Spiritual Competence for Mental Health Professionals

A Culturally Inclusive Perspective

Other Titles by the Author

Spiritual Competence for Mental Health Professionals

A Culturally Inclusive Perspective

Jacqueline Wallen

University of Maryland, USA

World Scientific

NEW JERSEY · LONDON · SINGAPORE · BEIJING · SHANGHAI · HONG KONG · TAIPEI · CHENNAI · TOKYO

Published by

World Scientific Publishing Co. Pte. Ltd.

5 Toh Tuck Link, Singapore 596224

USA office: 27 Warren Street, Suite 401-402, Hackensack, NJ 07601

UK office: 57 Shelton Street, Covent Garden, London WC2H 9HE

Library of Congress Cataloging-in-Publication Data

Names: Wallen, Jacqueline, author.

Title: Spiritual competence for mental health professionals :
a culturally inclusive perspective / Jacqueline Wallen.

Description: New Jersey : World Scientific, [2022] | Includes bibliographical references and index.

Identifiers: LCCN 2022001030 | ISBN 9789811243196 (hardcover) |
ISBN 9789811243202 (ebook for institutions) | ISBN 9789811243219 (ebook for individuals)

Subjects: LCSH: Psychotherapy--Religious aspects. | Psychotherapy patients--Religious life. |
Counseling--Religious aspects.

Classification: LCC RC489.S676 W35 2022 | DDC 616.89/14--dc23/eng/20220506

LC record available at https://lccn.loc.gov/2022001030

British Library Cataloguing-in-Publication Data

A catalogue record for this book is available from the British Library.

For any available supplementary material, please visit
https://www.worldscientific.com/worldscibooks/10.1142/12439#t=suppl

Desk Editor: Shaun Tan Yi Jie

Typeset by Stallion Press
Email: enquiries@stallionpress.com

About the Author

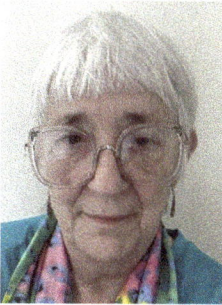

Dr. Jacqueline Wallen is Associate Professor Emerita in the Department of Family Science, School of Public Health, at University of Maryland at College Park, USA. She is a clinical and pastoral social worker with over 30 years of experience who provides spiritually grounded psychotherapy for all spiritual orientations as well as consultation to faith communities of all kinds. She holds a PhD and MA in Human Development from University of Chicago, USA, and a Master of Social Work degree from Catholic University of America, USA. She has previously published 3 books.

As a professor at the University of Maryland, Dr. Wallen designed, developed, and taught undergraduate and graduate courses on human services, program evaluation, family science, aging, substance abuse, and cultural competence. She won the University's Doris Sands Excellence in Teaching Award in 2014. As a clinical social worker, she retains a special interest in working with older adults and couples. Her clients go to her for help with a variety of issues, including life transitions, parenting or relationship difficulties, mental distress such as depression or anxiety, alcohol or drug problems, or a desire to resolve past traumas. Her primary modality is talk therapy (primarily cognitive behavioral and psychodynamic) but she is also trained in trauma treatment techniques such as EMDR and Somatic Experiencing. She has in-depth knowledge of 12-step programs such as AA, NA, and Alanon. She offers individual, couple, and family psychotherapy in her Silver Spring office and online using Zoom.

Contents

Chapter 1

Introduction and Overview

The purpose of this book is to contribute to the spiritual competence of mental health professionals across disciplines and international boundaries. It is impossible to write ethically about spiritual competence in mental health practice without addressing the long history of Anglo-European intellectual dominance and white supremacy in all areas of psychology, psychiatry, counseling, and social work. Most studies of spirituality and mental health have been conducted in North America or Europe and have had mostly Christian participants. The National Association of Social Workers has acknowledged that "Racism and white supremacy are ingrained within American institutions and systems and have therefore affected social work ideology and practice for generations" (National Association of Social Workers, 2020). In the book, *Crazy Like Us: The Globalization of the American Psyche*, author Ethan Watters showed how mental illnesses defined and popularized in America have become global at the cost of indigenous explanations and remedies for mental suffering. This book aims to counteract this bias by maintaining a more inclusive frame of reference with respect to spirituality and mental health, including, as much as possible, professional perspectives from a range of countries.

The concept of spiritual competence in clinical practice, as used here, means more than openness and the ability to work effectively with clients of divergent spiritual or religious perspectives. It also means having the knowledge and the tools to support clients' spiritual development as it affects their mental health and well-being. The developmental model used in this book is holistic, meaning that it views the individual as a whole — body, mind, and spirit — and is concerned with all three as they affect mental health. Another, unfortunately much more unwieldy, term often used for this perspective is "biopsychosocial-spiritual". This book draws on an international base of theory and research and acknowledges the global trend toward challenging the dominance of Western and Eurocentric paradigms for mental illness and mental health care. Discussion questions, exercises, and resources are presented at the end of each chapter.

Readers are cautioned not to stereotype individuals, families, or groups based on the descriptions of religious or spiritual orientations, beliefs, and practices described in this book or elsewhere. The risk of stereotyping as a result of cultural competence education or training has been noted but has not received a great deal of research attention (Buchtel, 2014). The same risk is present with spiritual competence training. Having a basic grasp of some major types of religious and spiritual belief is essential to a spiritually competent mental health practice. On the other hand, the cursory descriptions offered here are just the beginning of spiritual competence and there is no substitute for respectful inquiry, careful listening, and client-specific research to fully understand a client's spiritual issues and resources.

Certain wording choices in this book also deserve explanation. One has to do with the use of the terms "client" and "patient". English-speaking social workers and counselors tend to use the term "client" while those with medical training such as psychiatrists and psychiatric nurses tend to use the term "patient". Psychologists sometimes use one and sometimes the other, depending on their orientation. Mental health professionals in many other countries also differ among themselves in which term they use. In this book, we will use "client" unless we are directly quoting a source that uses "patient". A second has to do with naming the divinity in theistic religions. Every attempt is made in this book to show respect for all religious and spiritual orientations. When a monotheistic religion is discussed, the name of its God, Divinity, or Deity is capitalized as is done by the religion itself. When discussing the Jewish religion, the words G-d, or Holy One, are used to honor the Jewish tradition of not committing the holy name to writing. This originated to prevent it from being erased or disposed of disrespectfully.[1] The

---

[1] In Buddhism, a similar respect is shown for writings that contain the teachings of Buddha, though Buddha is not considered a deity, as well as for commentaries on his teachings and Buddhist liturgies. To prevent these texts from being disrespected, those who handle them are instructed to have clean hands and respectful minds. They are stored in clean and elevated places and disposed of ritually.

disclaimer relates to the case examples I have used. The case examples presented to illustrate theories, concepts, and interventions are either factual and known to the public, cited in the scholarly literature, or fictionalized composites of my clinical experience and observations with all identifying information removed or altered.

Chapter 2, "The Cultural Context of Science and Spirituality in Mental Health Care", shows how spiritual healing and mental health care have intertwined and diverged in various ways over time as shaped by their changing social and cultural contexts. It is only in relatively recent human history that a distinction has been made between the two and the trend toward reconciling the two has been even more recent. The effects of colonialism and neocolonialism on mental health care in non-Western countries are described and the concept of cultural relativism is presented and discussed. The concept of spiritual competence is introduced.

Chapter 3, "What is Spirituality", takes on the difficult task of defining spirituality and reviews differences among societies and cultures in the way that spirituality is conceptualized. Spirituality is defined, for the purpose of this book, as a "concern about, a search for, or a striving for understanding and relatedness to the transcendent" (Hill *et al.*, 2001). Dimensions of spirituality as reflected in words and phrases used to refer to it are: faith or beliefs, asking the big questions, moral and ethical values, disciplines or practices, character strengths or virtues, the pursuit of higher meaning, a transcendent experience, connection to the whole/diminishing of ego, and a brain-based cognitive, emotional, or somatic state. Spirituality can be secular and is a broader concept than religion, which is an institutionalized form of spirituality. The term spirituality is used for both in this book, except when citing an author who makes a deliberate distinction between the two.

Chapter 4, "Religions", describes the central beliefs of major world religions and common elements of local indigenous or folk religions. These include the Abrahamic religions, the major Dharmic Eastern religions, the nontheistic Eastern religions, the animistic religions, indigenous or folk religions, the occult, and new religious movements. Negative religious behavior such as religious abuse, religious prejudice and persecution, and violent religious extremism are discussed in detail. The importance of learning more about a client's religion by visiting websites related to the client's religion or religious organization, or reading articles or books about the religion, is stressed. Cultural humility is an important part of this process, but it is also important to be alert to possible negative influences of a client's or family's religious involvement.

Chapter 5, "Spirituality and Human Development", presents a holistic perspective on human development that integrates various stage theories of human development to show how social, psychological, and spiritual development influence one another. The development of a secure attachment to a parenting figure is emphasized as a foundation for healthy development in all three dimensions. Caveats are also given regarding the utility of stage theories. While they can be useful in alerting the clinician to potential client issues and resources, their linear organization is inconsistent with real-life developmental processes. Individual development occurs in fits and starts, is shaped by external events as much as internal timetables, does not necessarily move through stages in the order conceptualized by developmental theorists, and may include characteristics of more than one stage at once.

Chapter 6, "Spirituality and Mental Health", points out that while research generally shows a negative relationship between spirituality and mental illness, the relationship is complex and is not the same across all diagnostic categories. Because particular beliefs and practices may differ in their effects on mental health, spiritual orientations that create psychological stress are described. Religious fundamentalism as a barrier to the use of mental health services is analyzed.

Chapter 7, "Ethical Issues in Spiritual Competence", discusses the fact that because the concept of spiritual competence only emerged as an aspect of clinical competence in the past several decades, it is only implied in the ethical codes of most mental health professions. This chapter observes that clearer guidelines and more comprehensive professional education are needed. Standards for cultural competence that are included in the ethical codes of those professional associations that do have them are presented, along with criteria for evaluating professional education programs. Typical ethical issues and legal-ethical conflicts that arise in spiritually based psychotherapy are noted and a decision-making model is described. The ethical implications of transference and countertransference are discussed.

Chapter 8, "Assessing Spiritual Orientations, Needs, and Goals", provides a rationale for exploring clients' spiritual needs and issues and guidelines for integrating spiritual assessment into the overall assessment process. It also emphasizes the importance of self-awareness for mental health professionals and suggestions for including self-assessment in graduate train-ing programs. Commonly used methods and protocols for spiritual assess-ment are presented and spiritual issues and struggles are explored. The difficulty of distinguishing between psychosis and spiritual emergencies is noted and guidelines for assessment are presented. Common types of harm-ful belief and practice are described, including spiritually based abuse. Spiritual assessment is viewed as an ongoing process to be carried out throughout the treatment process.

Chapter 9, "Spiritually Competent Treatment", explores the boundaries of spiritually competent care and describes a range of spiritually inclusive and faith-based approaches to providing spiritually competent care. Tools that can be used across the range of client spiritual orientations are suggested. Helpful responses to spiritual crises or emergencies are described and the pros and cons of medication in these circumstances are analyzed. The use of psy-choactive or hallucinogenic substances as precipitators of or treatment for spiritual crises is examined.

Chapter 10, "Age and Stage-Related Issues and Interventions", is con-cerned with how to select age- and stage-appropriate interventions for indi-viduals and families over the life cycle. The importance of addressing past or current trauma at all ages is emphasized and end-of-life issues are addressed.

Chapter 11, "Professional Considerations", covers issues related to clini-cal supervision and referral, consultation, and collaboration with other pro-fessionals, including clergy and healers or spiritual leaders outside the professional structure of the Western medical system or formal licensing structure. Best practices for interacting with clergy and congregations are outlined. Considerations for ethical practice in faith-based organizations are reviewed.

Chapter 12, "Where Do We Go from Here?", suggests globally applica-ble directions for the improvement of spiritual competence in mental health care. They include decolonizing mental health and mental health care, pro-moting holistic definitions of mental health, advancing the evidence-based research base, integrating spirituality into professional practice and training, and working with clergy and faith-based communities.

Chapter 2

The Cultural Context of Science and Spirituality in Mental Health Care

"Religion and healing have been intertwined since earliest recorded history. Throughout history the role of the priest and the physician have overlapped frequently and have in many cultures been difficult to separate. For most of human history, there was no distinction at all between the two roles." (Thielman, 1998, p.4).

For most of human history, spiritual and religious healers and/or institutions have been responsible for the care of the mentally ill. In fact, the concept of mental illness is itself a relatively new one. Mental health and mental illness have been defined and viewed differently at different points in time. Mental illness has been viewed through a supernatural lens through most of human history and still is in many healing traditions. While humans, since the earliest times, have gathered, analyzed, and used information about their world, science as we know it today was a relatively late development in human history and has often been resisted by religious authorities. Psychiatry as a scientific discipline did not begin to emerge until the 19th century (Scull, 2015), and even then, faith-based organizations and religious groups were the primary caregivers, apart from families, of the seriously mentally ill. Over the centuries, spiritual or religious explanations and treatment for mental illness have sometimes been embraced and sometimes rejected by scientific authorities. The concept of "divine madness" has been a part of many cultures and religions. Divine madness refers to non-normative behavior that would otherwise be considered a sign of mental illness but that is, instead, a form of religious ecstasy or a deliberate teaching strategy. For our purposes, the current World Health Organization definition (2018) is probably the most useful:

> Health is a state of complete physical, mental, and social well-being and not merely the absence of disease or infirmity. An important implication of this definition is that mental health is more than just the absence of mental disorders or disabilities. … (It is) a state of well-being in which an individual realizes his or her own abilities, can cope with the normal stresses of life, can work productively and is able to make a contribution to his or her community.

Studies of clients receiving mental health services indicate that they see a connection between their spirituality and their mental health. A study of recipients of California public mental health services (Yamada *et al.*, 2020) found that 80% agreed or strongly agreed that spirituality was important to their mental health. The American Psychiatric Association (2018) defines mental illnesses as:

> Health conditions involving changes in emotion, thinking or behavior (or a combination of these). Mental illnesses are associated with distress and/or problems functioning in social, work or family activities.

The National Institute for Mental Health (n.d.) estimates that nearly one in five adults in the U.S. suffers from a mental illness. Only 5.2% suffer from a serious mental illness, however. Mental illnesses, or disorders, can range in severity from very mild to extremely severe, depending upon level of distress and degree of disturbance in functioning. Severity is an important factor in how societies respond to mental illness and different cultures have different standards for judging severity. There is diversity of opinion even within present-day Western medical culture. Zimmerman, Morgan, & Stanton (2018) point out that there are no general guidelines in the present-day Diagnostic and Statistical Manual of Mental Disorders (DSM-5) for characterizing a mental disorder as mild, moderate, or severe. Instead, the criteria vary from one disorder to another.

Lenski's paradigm (Nolan & Lenski, 2014), which is based on the premise that a society's primary technology shapes their social structure and culture, including their spiritual perspective, is used as a framework for the following discussion of religions, with the addition of one more category — post-industrial societies. Lenski's framework is helpful for organizing information about the relationship between spirituality and mental illness over time. A major problem with typologies like Lenski's is that they have, for the most part, originated in North America, Europe, or the British Isles and are therefore characterized by an implicit ethnocentric bias. Societies that more closely resemble these Western societies are often treated as more evolved because they emerged later in history. It is true that societies tend to change over time in fairly predictable ways, but this does not mean that later forms of social organization or religion are necessarily "more evolved" than earlier ones. In fact, many historically earlier religions still persist and continue to change today, and virtually all contemporary religions have incorporated elements of the religions that preceded them. To counteract the inherent bias toward modern Western societies, cultural anthropologists have long advocated "cultural relativism", which means that other cultures should be viewed in their own terms and not judged by standards of another culture. Another term, used in discussions of cultural competence, is "cultural humility". The concept of cultural humility was introduced by Tervalon & Murray-Garcia in 1998 to counteract the implication that cultural competence was a state that could be attained. They preferred the term cultural humility because it implied a lifelong process of learning and a respect for marginalized cultures. In this chapter we will look at the history of the relationship between spirituality and mental illness care but we do not intend to imply that religious or spiritual approaches that evolved later are necessarily superior to earlier ones.

2.1 Magico-religious healing

Modern, literate societies (societies with a written language) account for less than 1% of the human societies that have ever existed. The overwhelming majority of humans lived in **pre-literate** societies or what the anthropologist, Robert Redfield (1947), called "folk societies". These small, homogeneous societies rely on **hunting**, **gathering**, and perhaps some **subsistence farming** for their survival. They are typically nomadic or partially nomadic because their hunting and gathering eventually deplete local food and game resources, requiring them to seek out new areas in which to obtain food. They are organized around matrilineal or patrilineal kinship clans which they often believe are mystically related to a spirit being, generally a plant or animal on which they depend for food. Their animistic religious practices are aimed at worshiping and ensuring the proliferation of the totem animal or plant. Because all members of these societies must forage daily for their food, they lack enough surplus to support other kinds of specialized roles, with one exception. The exception is the, usually part-time, role of the folk healer or traditional healer, often referred to in Western writings as a shaman (Eliade, 2020), derived from the Siberian Tungu tribe word meaning "one who knows". Burger & Fristoe (2018) estimate that approximately ten million hunter-gatherers still exist today. While the earliest hunting and gathering societies were often isolated from other societies, today almost all of them have, to some extent, been affected by colonization and exposed to present-day culture and technology. Objections have been raised to the use of the word shaman as a generic term used by non-indigenous people to refer to the healers of pre-literate or modern indigenous societies. Penelope (2019) cautions that the term is only one of a number of terms that various indigenous languages have used to designate these healers and argues that the use of the world shaman as an umbrella term subtly reinforces the religious superiority of the West. She asks why we do not call them priests or, for that matter, why we don't call imams priests. Furthermore, she notes that the term shaman is racially charged since it implies primitivity and most indigenous healers/priests have been persons of color. She quotes Pharo (2011), who said:

> The paradigmatic post-colonial reduction of many indigenous religious system to "shamanism" has created an impoverished view of religions that are no less complex and sophisticated than the so-called "Great Traditions".

The **traditional healer** is someone, male, female, or transgendered, who possesses a body of tribal lore, passed down orally, concerning healing practices and the healing properties of local plants. Also, many native healers are believed to have special access to the spirit world, which they contact by entering into an altered state of consciousness, assisted by drumming, drugs, or other aids. During the trance, they negotiate with the spirits, asking them to cure the illness for which help was sought. Usually the cause of the illness, according to the spirits, is the violation of some tribal taboo and the individual and/or the entire community are required to make reparations of some kind. The earliest known archeological evidence of shamanism was the burial site of a shaman, who may have been a woman, that dated back to over 30,000 years ago (Tedlock, 2005).

Another diagnosis that was made by folk healers in many early societies is referred to in Western anthropology and modern neo-shamanists such as Harner

(1990) as "**soul loss**". Johansen (2003) has argued that this term is inaccurate because people in early folk societies did not believe in the existence of a single soul within each person (though they did have other concepts to represent the non-physical aspects of the self). Still, they believed that parts of a person's vital being could be left behind or seized by **demons**, especially when a person was extremely stressed or frightened. Fadiman (1998) has documented the tragic death of a Laotian Hmong refugee child with epilepsy whose American doctors failed to take into account the fact that her family believed her to be suffering from soul loss rather than a medical condition. As a result, they did not follow the doctors' instructions and the child's seizures worsened until she died. The condition the term soul loss refers to would today be called "posttraumatic stress disorder (PTSD)". The process used by indigenous healers, both in the past and today, of treating PTSD has been referred to by anthropologists as "soul retrieval". Gonzales (2012) describes the healing of soul loss in the indigenous traditions of Mesoamerica, referring to it as "susto" (a Mexican term) or "displacement of an animating force". Mesoamerican folk healers, or curanderos, still often engage in rituals involving raw eggs, sweeping the body with brooms made from local plants, and sweat lodges to treat soul loss (Figure 2.1).

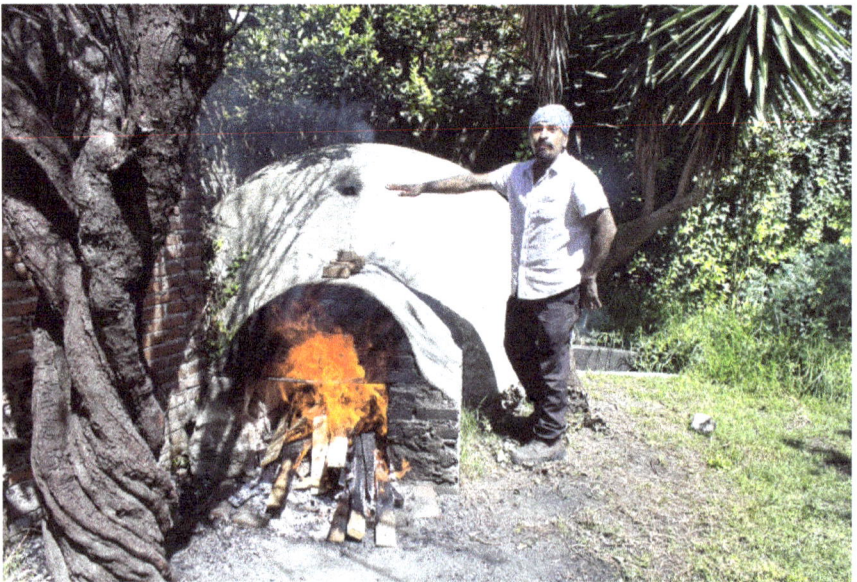

Figure 2.1.   An indigenous healer standing next to his sweat lodge.

In their review of the literature on indigenous or traditional healers, Struthers *et al.* (2004) highlight the prominence placed on the spiritual world and supernatural forces in indigenous healing, but they also underscore its holistic foundations and its emphasis on community well-being and social connections. Indigenous healers invoke spirits and the supernatural in their healing rituals while psychotherapists typically do not. Yet de Rios (2002), a medical anthropologist and licensed psychotherapist, has studied traditional Peruvian folk healers and describes how therapists and folk healers often use similar techniques, including:

- The power of suggestion or, in psychotherapeutic lingo, hypnosis. Both the healer/therapist and the patient/client enter into altered states of consciousness, reducing resistance and empowering the patient/client.
- Behavior modification to alter dysfunctional behaviors.
- Cognitive restructuring to restructure beliefs and eliminate negative self-talk.
- Supporting empowerment and sense of self-efficacy.
- Herbal remedies for depression and anxiety.

2.2 Distinction between the spiritual and the secular

By around 10,000 BCE, societies in the fertile regions of Mesopotamia (Iraq, Kuwait, Turkey, and Syria) began to domesticate livestock and develop metal tools for farming. This has been referred to as the "Neolithic revolution" or the "agricultural revolution". Gradually, and at different times and rates, **horticultural** (small-scale farming) and **pastoral** (herding) societies developed in other parts of the world as well. Horticulture is particularly suited to hot, humid climates. Though horticultural societies are larger and more settled than hunting and gathering ones, they may still be semi-nomadic because their farming methods are rudimentary and may gradually deplete the plant nutrients in their local soil. Their belief systems are generally polytheistic, and their religious practices focus on rain and crops. Pastoral, or herding, societies depend heavily on domesticated animals for their food supply. They also can be larger, and may be settled, nomadic, or semi-nomadic, depending on the abundance of grazing resources. Many pastoral societies developed monotheistic religions with deities that were involved in human affairs. Both horticultural and pastoral arrangements support the accumulation of enough food surplus to permit the emergence of some specialized roles not directly related to the acquisition of food. A degree of social stratification exists in such societies. Shamanism is accorded a higher status and eventually becomes an elite priesthood in which the concept of spirits is coupled with the idea of gods or a God. Winkelman (1986) has used the term "**magico-religious practitioner**" to refer to healers that have attributes of both shamans and priests. Pastoral societies may be tribal- or clan-based while horticultural societies typically consist of extended family units. Horticulture is still practiced successfully in tropical forest areas in the Amazon Basin and on mountain slopes in South and Central America, as well as low population density areas of North Africa, Central Africa, Southeast Asia, and Melanesia. Pastoralism remains a way of life in many parts of the world. Mbow *et al.* (2019) estimate that 200–500 million people live in pastoral communities and that there are pastoral communities in 75% of all countries.

Mental illness in these societies is still often viewed as demon possession and one of the earliest documented surgical procedures is the drilling or scraping of one or more holes in the skull to release the supposed demon(s). André (2017) has thoroughly reviewed the literature on this process, which is now called trepanation or trephination and which dates back to 7,000–10,000 years ago. He notes that it was still used in some parts of Africa and Oceania (a large collection of islands in the Pacific) well into the 20th century. He also points out that there was a resurgence in the use of trepanning in the Western world in the 1960s and 1970s, particularly among some groups interested in altering the mind and expanding consciousness, and notes that trepanning is still being performed in some facilities in North America and Europe. The *British Medical Journal* has warned that websites exist that promote trepanning for several conditions, including depression and chronic fatigue syndrome, and has cautioned against self-trepanning, rates of which have risen because most doctors are not willing to do trepanning for these conditions. The journal notes that while trepanation is relatively safe when performed by a skilled neurosurgeon, it is very risky when people perform it on themselves (BMJ, 2000). It is interesting that a procedure that is not totally different from trepanation is now being tested in the U.S. Bernstein (2021) describes an experimental treatment for drug addiction that involves cutting two "nickel-sized" holes in a patient's brain and stimulating the brain with metal-tipped electrodes. This procedure has also been used for Parkinson's disease, epilepsy, and a few other intractable conditions.

2.3 Roots of modern medicine

Advances in technological development led to farming on a much larger scale beginning around 3,000 BCE, producing sufficient grain to feed domestic animals. The amount of food a single family could produce increased drastically and the excess could be sold or bartered, which eventually led to moneyed economies. Land ownership became the basis for wealth and resulted in more settled communities. Because of the food surplus, those who did not farm could do other kinds of work, which supported the growth of larger and more complex societies with more occupational specialization. Artisans and tradespeople began to gather in **urban centers**, creating the first small cities. **Agrarian** societies are typically rigidly stratified, however, so that most people did not experience an improvement in their food supply. Over time, medicine and the priesthood became separate institutions with their own bodies of knowledge and educational facilities, usually in city centers, though mental illness was still attributed by both to gods, demons, or spirits. In patriarchal societies men have more power and authority than women and they alone can own and control property. As a result, male offspring are highly valued while female offspring are not. Most of the major world religions originated in agrarian times so that their foundational texts reflect the patriarchal assumptions and values of the times. Gregg (2005) has argued that the extreme social inequality based on ownership of property in agrarian societies was what led to a belief in the Evil Eye, which still persists in some traditional Mediterranean societies. Because property was so important and so unequally distributed, people at all economic levels feared envy and developed protective rituals to avoid being cursed with the Evil Eye by others. Many illnesses, including mental illness, were attributed to the Evil Eye.

Different scholars report different timelines, but it seems safe to say that as early as the 2nd century BCE, the **Ayurvedic** school of medicine had emerged in India, beginning with medical references in sacred texts such as the Vedas (Narayanaswamy, 1981). Mental illness was diagnosed by observation and pulse palpation to identify and guide in balancing the relative strengths of three different body energies (Kumar & Shrivastava, 2000). Mental health resulted from a balance of these energies and personality characteristics were thought to be determined by their relative strengths. Imbalances resulting in mental illness were thought to be caused by diet, disrespect toward the gods, or "mental shock due to excessive fear or joy" (*ibid*, p. 1).

Ayurvedic medicine advocates a healthy lifestyle and is still practiced in many countries and cultures today. In India, Ayurvedic practitioners can receive a bachelor's degree in Ayurvedic medicine and, like medical doctors, are licensed by the state. Again, scholars differ in their estimates, but somewhere during that same general time period, Chinese medicine developed the medical system of **acupuncture**, also based on balancing energies and encouraging the free flow of Qi, or life force energy, through the body. In traditional Chinese acupuncture, Qi is made up of complementary forces called yin and yang. Yin energy refers to darkness, femininity, passivity, and receptiveness. Yang energy refers to brightness, masculinity, activity, and assertiveness. Acupuncture treatments are used to restore balance as necessary. Techniques included herbal remedies and stimulation through applying pressure, burning dried herbs, or pricking the skin with a needle along what came to be called energy meridians. Further developments in acupuncture included treatments for balancing the interactions among five basic elements: wood (anger), fire (joy), earth (worry), metal (sadness), and water (fear). Physical and mental illnesses were thought to be a result of imbalances in these elements. Acupuncture is still widely used and at present there are many accredited acupuncture schools in the U.S. and other countries. There is considerable research evidence that an acupuncture detoxification protocol for drug addiction developed by Michael Smith (NADA, n.d.) is effective and the World Health Organization has accepted acupuncture as a treatment for drug abuse (Motlagh *et al.*, 2016).

While Indian and Chinese medicine were taking shape, Egyptian physicians were beginning to investigate physical or "natural" causes of mental illness, though they still believed in supernatural causes of mental illness as well. They invented a term to describe mental illness in women — **hysteria** — which meant "wandering uterus". Many authors (e.g., Tasca *et al.*, 2012) have pointed out that this diagnosis and the methods of treating it reflected patriarchal views of women as weak, vulnerable to mental disorders, and ruled by their sexuality and reproductive function. Hippocrates, the Greek physician who is often considered the founder of Western medicine, was born in the 5th century BCE. He viewed human beings as consisting of both a body and a soul but did not believe that illness resulted from magical or supernatural causes. He believed, like the Egyptians, that it had natural, or physical, causes. He and his followers distinguished their approach from that of the temple healers, who claimed miraculous cures based on the use of spells, charms, incantations, and purification rites aimed at inducing divine intervention (Scull, 2015). In contrast to the existing Hellenic view that the heart was the seat of emotions, Hippocrates located them in the brain. Like Indian and Chinese physicians, Hippocrates stressed balance but, for him, the balance to be sought related to **four body fluids or "humors"**. The four humors were: blood (activity), yellow bile (anger), black bile (melancholia), and phlegm (apathy). The concept of humoral imbalance continued to be used to explain mental illness throughout the Middle Ages and humoral treatments were applied even into the 19th century. For example, bloodletting was used to treat the manic phase of bipolar disorder because the condition was thought to result from too much blood. Bloodletting was also used to treat depression, thought to be caused by an excess of black bile, along with purging (with emetics and/or laxatives) and exercise. Despite Hippocrates' work, Greek folk medicine still attributed mental illness to demons or curses of the gods and many people turned to priests and temples for healing. Hippocrates' theory of the humors continued to be influential in the 2nd century, when the Greek physician Galen was born. Galen studied at many different medical schools and was greatly influenced by Hippocrates' ideas. He described a syndrome that he called Lypē, which resembled our current conception of an anxiety disorder (Mattern, 2016). Like Hippocrates, Galen attributed mental illness to natural rather than supernatural causes.

Christianity in Europe in the first few centuries incorporated many of the old pagan beliefs attributing mental illness to the work of demons. It also stood in the way of the advancement of medicine as a scientific discipline because of its prohibitions against the dissection of human corpses. Care for the mentally ill was provided either by families in the local community, or by monasteries and church-run hospitals, in which care was mostly benevolent but custodial rather than rehabilitative. By the 8th century, sophisticated hospitals were being developed in the Arab world, based on the ancient Greek texts. There, the dissection of corpses was allowed and doctors contributed important new ideas in the areas of pediatrics, anatomy, and surgery. Physicians and hospitals in the Arabic-Islamic world were known to offer treatment for the mentally ill, and some hospitals even offered music therapy (Koenig, 2005). Koetschet (2016) describes three examples of mental illness that were treated in Arabic hospitals: **epilepsy, delirium, and melancholy**. Though physicians differed in what they defined as melancholy, the most eminent physician of the time was Avicenna, a Persian, whose description had much in common with the contemporary view of bipolar disorder. Hospitals were used both to confine and to treat mental patients, and clinical experiments were actually carried out in some Arabic hospitals. Koetschet tells of a controlled experiment in which a physician named Al-Razi treated one group of patients with bloodletting and left another alone, then observed the result to determine its effectiveness.

Bromberg has asserted that:

> The tangled strands of psychotherapy during this vast period (the first mil-
> lennium of Christianity) can be separated into two main streams — rational
> therapy with an accent on bodily hygiene, and mystical faith healing under
> the canopy of the Christian, Moslem, and Jewish faiths. (Bromberg, 1975,
> p. 23).

But Rider (2011) disagrees, arguing that these were not necessarily distinct trends, since priests and doctors often agreed on treatments. Even today, religious or supernatural explanations of mental illness are common in predominantly agrarian societies. In India, for example, where there is only one psychiatrist for every 400,000 people, most people with substance abuse problems, severe depression, and psychotic disorders turn to faith healers and temples for help (Kennedy, 2010). In Europe, throughout the Middle Ages (roughly 500 to 1500 CE), healing powers were claimed for relics of Catholic saints and healing for physical and mental illness was sought in shrines and churches, where practices included exorcism or the casting out of demons. At the same time, Greek humoral theories were reintroduced into Europe by way of translations of Arabic texts.

England's first mental hospital, **Bethlehem Hospital**, was founded in 1257. Its patients were largely poor and had no one else to look after them. It became a symbol of the overcrowding and brutal treatment often found in the "lunatic asylums" of Europe and North America. The word "bedlam", used to denote noise and chaos, was derived from the name Bethlehem. Bromberg (1975) cautions that such maltreatment was not necessarily the norm in Europe. Many institutions that cared for the mentally ill were humane and kind. European-influenced ideas about hospital care for the mentally ill gradually spread to other countries. The invention of the printing press in Europe in the 1400s permitted medical knowledge, such as it was, to be more widely disseminated, though the scientific method was not yet a significant influence on beliefs about mental illness. Colonialism was also responsible for spreading Western ideas about mental illness to other parts of the world, though the largest contiguous empire in world history was created by Mongolian pastoral herders under Genghis Khan in the 13th and 14th centuries A.D. The Mongols colonized large parts of Asia, Iran, Russia, Eastern Europe, China, and many other countries. Though Genghis Khan was an animist who believed in shamanism, he encouraged religious freedom. Buddhism, Islam, and Christianity were all practiced in the Mongolian Empire. Toward the end of the 15th century, the discovery of new shipping routes enabled European countries to explore and colonize large parts of the American and Asian continents. Colonization occurs when one country takes political control of another country, populating it with settlers, and exploiting it economically. It brings into contact differing cultures of unequal power and results in oppressive doctrines of racial and/or ethnic inferiority and superiority. European colonial powers generally endeavored to suppress or eliminate indigenous religions and often used mental institutions to silence dissidents (e.g., Keller, 2007; Rajpal, 2020; Yoo, 2016). During that same period, Islamic forces created what was called the Ottoman Empire, which encompassed large parts of the Middle East and Eastern Europe. It was governed from Constantinople, now called Istanbul. Also, around the same time, Russia was creating its own empire by expanding northward and to either side. By the mid-17th century, the Dutch East India company had established a colony in Cape Town, South Africa. One of the largest colonial empires was established by the Japanese in the western Pacific and East Asian regions.

2.4 Science vs. spirituality in mental health care

Between the 17th and 19th centuries, Europe and North America experienced what has been called a "scientific revolution" in which a reliance on science and reason gradually eroded the belief in religious authority and tradition.

This period was called the "Enlightenment". Knowledge based on empirical research began to displace the ancient Greek humoral theories, though many earlier medical practices such as bloodletting persisted. The development of manufacturing industries in Britain, Europe, and the U.S. beginning around the end of the 18th century led to what has been called "**the industrial revolution**". Industrialization gradually spread to other parts of the world, though many societies remain primarily agriculture-based with developing industrial economies. Satellite data have shown that as recently as 2005, 40% of the Earth's surface was still used for agriculture (Owen, 2005).

As societies industrialize, populations become more concentrated in cities and their outskirts. While local communities and extended families are important sources of support for the mentally ill in agrarian societies, these ties may be weakened in industrial societies as geographic mobility increases. Educational and medical centers flourish and a belief in science may replace superstition for many. The 17th and 18th centuries in Europe were labelled the "Age of Enlightenment" or "Age of Reason". Value was placed on science and the scientific method while traditional and religious authority became less influential. During this time, there was considerable interest in the mind, both as a physical structure and as a process of thought. By the late 18th century, Cullen had proposed the idea that nerve impulses were responsible for mental illness (the neurosis theory of disease) (Bromberg, 1975). As more was learned about the brain and its relationship to thoughts and feelings, supernatural theories of mental illness fell into disrepute. Around the time of Cullen, Philippe Pinel in France advocated for the humane treatment of the mentally ill and argued for what he called "**moral treatment**", which was a combination of psychological and religious or moral techniques such as conversation, recreation, and exercise. Dorothea Dix, an advocate of the moral method of treatment, was deeply disturbed by the inhumane conditions in U.S. asylums and helped establish 32 state mental hospitals based on that method. The moral approach spread to other countries as well, improving conditions for the mentally ill in hospitals. By the 19th century, humanitarian reforms were introduced in the asylums. Standards for care were established and attempts to treat patients with various forms of therapy began to replace the goal of simply containing them. Stimulated by the new field of psychoanalysis, a perspective Thielman (*op. cit.*) calls "**radical secularism**" emerged in the field of mental health care. Psychology, which had previously been a branch of philosophy, emerged as a field in its own right, with graduate schools and professional organizations of its own. Mental illness was "**medicalized**", meaning that it came to be viewed by experts as a medical problem rather than a spiritual one. The term "mental illness" began to replace the word "madness" (Scull, 2015). By the mid-19th century, a specialty known as neurology had begun to study disorders of the nervous system and psychotherapeutic techniques such as hypnosis were being used by physicians in hospitals and clinics. Nevertheless, the institutions that provided care for the mentally ill remained overcrowded and little progress was made in treatment. By the end of the 19th century, however, Freud's "**psychoanalysis**" had been adopted by many doctors, and outpatient treatment, at least for the wealthy, had become an option. At the same time, faith healers were still popular, and Mary Baker Eddy, the founder of the Christian Science religion, had started a non-medical college for Christian Science healers. William James was an advocate for the "**mind-cure movement**", which stressed the healing power of positive emotions and beliefs. Duclow (2002) summarizes the features of mind-cure, according to James:

- Suggestion, or using the power of ideas to heal (e.g., affirmations, visualization, meditation).
- Letting go, or surrendering our attempts to heal ourselves through the power of our will.
- Mobilizing the healing energies of the subconscious.

Mind-cure approaches have also been called the "New Thought Movement" and are integral to a variety of denominations and churches such as the Unity Church and the Divine Science Church. They also are at the core of many mind/body interventions such as meditation, relaxation and breathing techniques, yoga, hypnosis, and biofeedback.

Sigmund Freud was a contemporary of William James. His psychoanalytic method was based on free association on the part of the patient and dialogue between the patient and the physician. He considered religion an infantile way of thinking and reinforced the colonial belief that indigenous people were inferior beings whose thinking was similar to that of the mentally ill. His book on the subject, *Totem and Taboo* (1919), had the subtitle: *Resemblances between the Psychic Lives of Savages and Neurotics.* Freud's negative attitude toward spirituality and religion created a major split between psychotherapy and spiritual thought that persists among many scholars and clinicians today. **Behaviorism**, the other major school of psychology at the time, also contributed significantly to that rift. Behavioral psychologists declined to study or theorize about the inner psychological world, focusing only on empirically observable stimuli, behavioral responses, and positive or negative reinforcements. Both psychoanalysis and behaviorism were reductionist in the sense that they felt that behavior was shaped by a desire to satisfy basic biological needs.

In the 1930s, Carl Jung (2001) broke with psychoanalysis to assert that life has a spiritual purpose, and that spiritual experience is essential to psychological well-being. Around the same time, some theological schools in the U.S. and elsewhere began providing clinical training for their students. Many countries now have certificating bodies for **clinical pastoral education** and many universities now offer dual degrees in Divinity and a mental health profession. Abraham **Maslow** (1943) is often given credit for stimulating the development of the humanistic school of psychotherapy. Maslow distinguished between two kinds of needs. The first kind he called "deficiency needs". These were the basic needs that caused intrapsychic conflict in Freudian theory and that were rewarded and reinforced in behaviorism. The needs identified in the first four levels of Maslow's hierarchy of needs pyramid (Figure 2.2) were the ones he called deficiency needs, or d-needs.

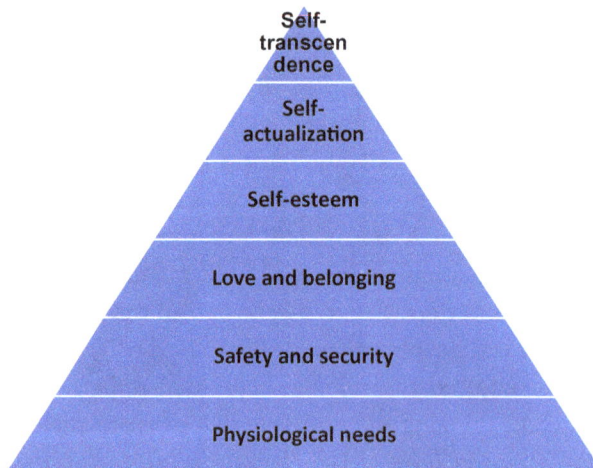

Figure 2.2. Maslow's hierarchy of needs.

The top triangle represents a being need, or b-need. Different needs predominate at different times and Maslow arranged needs in a hierarchy to indicate that lower-level needs must be satisfied before higher-level needs become motivators. Physiological needs such as hunger, thirst, sleep, and shelter have to do with survival and must be satisfied before other needs demand satisfaction. Once these have been met, safety and security become motivating needs. The next motivational level in Maslow's hierarchy is social needs — the need to be connected to other people through couple or family relationships, friendship, group membership, etc. Self-esteem needs have to do with the need for approval and recognition. Self-actualization is the full realization of one's creative, intellectual, psychological, and social potential. While this is the highest level shown in almost all graphic depictions of Maslow's hierarchy of needs, he actually added a sixth level later in his life (Koltko-Rivera, 2006). He called this level self-transcendence, or the need for communion with the transcendent. At this level, people identify with something greater than the individual self and often engage in service to others. He coined the term "transpersonal psychology" to indicate a psychological approach that included a focus on self-transcendence. Maslow (1964) used the term "**peak experience**" to refer to the highest level of experience — self-transcendence.

In 1946, Viktor Frankl, an Austrian psychiatrist and neurologist, developed a method of **existential** psychotherapy that he named "**logotherapy**" (1967). It was based on observations he had made while a prisoner in a German concentration camp during World War II. Frankl had observed that concentration camp prisoners who were able to find a positive purpose in life were the ones most apt to survive. He called his approach "existentialist" because, like the European existentialist philosophers of his time, he focused on the human search for meaning in the face of anxiety, suffering, and even death. He felt that finding meaning and purpose in life was the key to mental health. Frankl's views contradicted Maslow's concept of a hierarchy of needs because he argued that even when starving and mistreated, concentration camp prisoners continued to seek meaning in their lives. Frankl, in turn, has been accused of victim-blaming because his work can be read to imply that those who did not survive in concentration camps were somehow at fault, but others argue that this is a misinterpretation (Simon, 2020).

2.5 Reconciliation of science and religion

The 1960s saw the emergence of, using the term popularized by Daniel Bell (1974), "**post-industrial societies**". These are societies in which the service sector plays a bigger role in the economy than the manufacturing sector. Societies that experience significant technological advancement are eventually able to automate many of the functions that have been performed by manual laborers and the development of increasingly more sophisticated computers creates new businesses and markets. While the manufacturing sector produces physical items such as automobiles, appliances, or clothing, most of the products of the service sector are intangible. They include such services as warehousing and transportation, information processing, professional services, health care, research, recreation, and the arts. The U.S. was the first country to have more than 50% of its workers employed in the service sector. Other post-industrial societies include Japan and most of Europe. The transition to a post-industrial economy results in a decrease in working-class jobs and an increase of middle-class jobs requiring more formal education and more social skills.

The 1960s also marked the beginnings of the **"New Age" spiritual movement** in the West. The concept of New Age spirituality denotes a heterogeneous mix of spiritual beliefs and practices that gained prominence in the Western world, especially the U.S. and Great Britain, during the 1970s and continued to grow in the 80s and 90s. Some religious scholars call the emergence of this trend the "New Age Movement". The movement included aspects of many ancient, indigenous, Eastern, and occult traditions and was heavily influenced by what was called the Human Potential Movement in psychology. The **Human Potential Movement** encompassed a variety of spiritual and psychological techniques aimed at helping individuals reach their full potential. This movement, according to the Pew Research Foundation (Gecewicz, 2018), includes beliefs in reincarnation, astrology, psychics, and the presence of spiritual energy in objects such as lime mountains or trees. The Pew research found that roughly 60% of Americans accepted at least one of these beliefs, including many religiously unaffiliated persons. **Eastern philosophies and religions** began to be integrated into Western psychotherapeutic approaches during these same years. In his book, *Psychotherapy East and West* (1961), the Zen scholar Alan Watts contended that Buddhism could be thought of as a form of psychotherapy. Compton

(2012) has described some of the major Eastern concepts and practices that have influenced Western psychotherapy:

- A holistic perspective (body, mind, spirit)
- Belief in the illusory nature of the everyday world
- The practice of meditation
- An emphasis on the direct experience of the underlying unity of the cosmos
- Transcendence of self or ego
- Lack of distinction between the sacred and the secular

R. D. Laing, writing in the 1960s, was a strong defender of the **antipsychiatry movement** and deplored the dehumanizing conditions that prevailed in mental institutions at the time. Rather than pathologizing mental illness, he idealized it, and felt that with the proper support, it could be self-healing and even enable spiritual growth (Burston, 1998). His voice supported the argument for deinstitutionalization and contributed to the development of community mental health care, but because he ignored research on the neurochemical and genetic factors involved in mental illness and rejected outright the usefulness of psychotropic medication, his ideas have been largely discredited. The 1960s and 1970s have been called the "**psychedelic era**" (Pendergast & Pendergast, 2000, p. 129) because of the influence of psychedelic drugs on society, music, and art during those years. Hallucinogens derived from plants have been used in spiritual practice in many cultures over time, but in 1960 the Harvard psychiatrist Timothy Leary began conducting experiments to determine whether the hallucinogens psilocybin and LSD were effective adjuvant agents in psychotherapy. Over the past decade there has been a renewed interest in "psychedelic-assisted" psychotherapy for posttraumatic stress disorder, depression, and cancer-related anxiety but the research is still in its early stages and has not produced any definitive results.

Increasingly, the concept of "spiritual health" has been finding its way into research and practice in mental health care. Crisp has observed that scholarship has moved beyond what she calls the "Anglosphere" to include the perspectives of indigenous people. A number of authors have suggested extending the "**biopsychosocial**" model of health and mental health that is assumed by most mental health professions to a "**biopsychosocial-spiritual**" model that includes the spiritual dimension of well-being (Saad *et al.*, 2017; Verghese, 2008). Such a model would validate spiritual health as a legitimate concern in mental health care. Transpersonal psychology is a concept that emerged from Maslow's discussion of self-actualization and encompasses a variety of approaches. The term "transpersonal" is used to refer to "experiences in which the sense of identity or self extends beyond (trans) the individual or personal to encompass wider aspects of humankind, life, psyche, or cosmos" (Walsh & Vaughan, 1993). "Positive psychology" is a term coined by Seligman & Csikszentmihalyi (2000). It also concerns itself with self-actualization, or what Seligman has called "**flourishing**" rather than on diagnosing and treating mental illness. Peterson (2008) defines positive psychology as:

> A scientific approach to studying human thoughts, feelings, and behavior, with a focus on strengths instead of weaknesses, building the good in life instead of repairing the bad, and taking the lives of average people up to 'great' instead of focusing solely on moving those who are struggling up to 'normal'.

For Seligman (2011), flourishing has five elements: positive emotion, engagement in life and work, positive relationships, meaning in life and work, and accomplishments. Many positive psychologists stress the importance of spirituality as a factor that leads to increased individual happiness and well-being.

2.6 Cultural, religious, and spiritual competence

In colonial imperialism, a country conquers and rules over another region. Western colonial imperialism was, for the most part, gradually replaced by neocolonialism in the latter half of the 20th century. In neocolonialism, economic, political, cultural, or other pressures are used to control, influence, and exploit other countries. Watters (2010) argues that one result of **neocolonialism** has been that the Western mental health profession has had a remarkable global influence over the meaning and treatment of mental illness. Mental health professionals, mostly U.S.-trained, have created official, worldwide categories of mental disorder in the American Psychiatric

Association's *Diagnostic and Statistical Manual of Mental Disorders* and its clone, *The International Classification of Mental and Behavioral Disorders.* Watters says:

> In addition, American researchers and organizations run the premier scholarly journals and host top conferences in the fields of psychology and psychiatry. Western universities train the world's most influential clinicians and academics. Western drug companies dole out the funds for research and spend billions marketing medications for mental illnesses. Western-trained traumatologists rush in wherever war or natural disasters strike to deliver "psychological first aid", bringing with them their assumptions about how the mind becomes broken and how it is best healed (pp. 3–4).

"**Cultural relativism**" is a term coined by the anthropologist Franz Boas in 1887. It means viewing a person's beliefs or practices based on that person's own culture rather than our own. "**Ethnocentrism**" is a related term, first used by the sociologist Ludwig Gumplowicz (McCornack & Ortiz, 2017, p. 109), to refer to the view that the beliefs and practices of one's own culture are superior to those of other cultures. Cultural relativism gradually became the preferred perspective in anthropology but was not incorporated into mental health practice until much later. The term "cultural competence" was first used by Cross *et al.* (1989) at the Georgetown University Child Development Center. These authors defined **cultural competence** as:

> A set of congruent behaviors, attitudes, and policies that come together in a system, agency or among professionals and enable that system, agency or those professions to work effectively in cross-cultural situations.

Their focus was primarily on the cultural competence of organizations, and they identified five essential elements that contribute to cultural competence:

1. Valuing diversity.
2. Having the capacity for cultural self-assessment.
3. Being conscious of the dynamics inherent when cultures interact.
4. Having institutionalized culture knowledge.

5. Having developed adaptations to service delivery reflecting an under-standing of cultural diversity.

The Georgetown framework describes a continuum of cultural compe-tence with six stages:

1. **Cultural destructiveness**: Attitudes, policies, structures, and practices within a system or organization that are destructive to a cultural group.
2. **Cultural incapacity**: An inability to respond effectively to the needs, interests, and preferences of culturally and linguistically diverse groups.
3. **Cultural blindness**: An expressed philosophy of viewing and treating all people as the same.
4. **Cultural pre-competence**: Awareness of needs for growth in order to respond effectively to culturally and linguistically diverse populations.
5. **Cultural competence**: Acceptance and respect for cultural differences. Ability to respond effectively to culturally and linguistically diverse populations.
6. **Cultural proficiency**: Placing a high value on all cultures. A lifelong process of acquiring cultural knowledge and expertise with a commit-ment to educating others.

Cultural competence now is an important requirement in the ethical guidelines of many professional organizations and mental health treatment models. For example, in 2019 the U.S. Substance Abuse and Mental Health Services Administration published the Treatment Improvement Protocol (TIP): *Behavioral Health Services for American Indians and Alaska Natives*, which affirms the importance of honoring indigenous people's cultures and traditions, and provides guides for incorporating culturally responsive prac-tices. An important development in cultural competence has been the emer-gence of the concept of "**intersectionality**". Crenshaw (1989; 2017) pointed out that we all have multiple intersecting and overlapping social identities such as gender, caste, race, class, sexuality, religion, disability, physical appearance, and height. As a feminist, she pointed out that each of these identities confers a degree of advantage and/or disadvantage so that, for example, being a Black gay male couple is not the same as being a white gay female couple. Al'Uqdah *et al.* (2019) give the example of African American

Muslims, noting that they constitute 40% of the Muslims in the U.S., but are virtually absent from the research literature. They observe that this highlights the invisibility of people with intersecting marginal identities.

In recent years, religious competence has received attention as an important aspect of cultural competence. Whitley & Jarvis (2015) define religious competence as:

> Skills, practices, and orientations that recognize, explore, and harness patient religiosity to facilitate diagnosis, recovery, and healing. Religious competence involves the learning and deployment of generic competencies, including active listening and a nonjudgmental stance. It is also an overarching orientation, providing a safe place for discussion of religious issues and identities received in a humble, respectful, and empathetic manner.

Spiritual competence is only rarely discussed separately from religious competence in the professional literature. Hodge (2015) views spiritual competence as a continuing learning process characterized by an increasing or growing:

- awareness of one's own value-informed worldview along with its assumptions, limitations, and biases.
- empathic, strengths-based understanding of the client's spiritual worldview.
- ability to design and implement interventions that resonate with the client's spiritual worldview.

When authors refer explicitly to spiritual competence, they typically use the term "spiritual/religious competence" and sometimes an acronym such as "SRC" or "SORC". The distinction between religion and spirituality will be discussed in greater detail in the next chapter. Vieten *et al.* (2013) define spiritual and religious competence as:

> A subset of multicultural competencies, spiritual and religious competencies are defined as a set of attitudes, knowledge, and skills in the domains of spirituality and religion that every psychologist should have to effectively and ethically practice psychology, regardless of whether or not they conduct spiritually oriented psychotherapy (p. 5).

The 16 aspects of spiritual and religious competence that they identify apply not just to psychologists but to all mental health professionals (p. 7). They are:

1. Demonstrating empathy, respect, and appreciation for clients from diverse spiritual, religious, or secular backgrounds and affiliations.
2. Viewing spirituality and religion as important aspects of human diversity.
3. Being aware of how their own spiritual and/or religious background and beliefs may influence their clinical practice.
4. Learning about spiritual and/or religious beliefs, communities, and practices that are important to their clients.
5. Understanding that spirituality and religion can be viewed as overlapping, yet distinct, constructs.
6. Awareness that clients may have experiences that are consistent with their spirituality or religion yet may be difficult to differentiate from psychopathological symptoms.
7. Recognizing that spiritual and/or religious beliefs, practices, and experiences develop and change over the lifespan.
8. Knowledge about spiritual and/or religious resources and practices that research indicates may support mental health.
9. Ability to identify spiritual and religious experiences, practices, and beliefs that may be harmful to mental health.
10. Ability to identify legal and ethical issues related to spirituality and/or religion that may surface when working with clients.
11. Ability to conduct empathic and effective psychotherapy with clients from diverse spiritual and/or religious backgrounds, affiliations, and levels of involvement.
12. Inquiring about spiritual and/or religious background, experience, practices, attitudes and beliefs as a standard part of understanding a client's history.
13. Helping clients explore and access their spiritual and/or religious strengths and resources.
14. Ability to identify and address spiritual and/or religious problems in clinical practice and make referrals when necessary.
15. Remaining current on research and professional developments regarding spirituality and religion specifically related to clinical practice, assessing their own spiritual and religious competence on a continuing basis.

16. Recognizing the limits of their qualifications and competence in the spiritual and/or religious domains, seeking consultation and further training when necessary.

In this chapter we have examined the history of the evolution of the diverse range of current attitudes regarding the relationship between spirituality in its various manifestations and the provision of care for the mentally ill. Scientific theories of mental illness are a relatively new development in human history and magical, spiritual, or religious treatments are still common in many parts of the world today. While the emergence of medical and psychological explanations for mental illness was initially accompanied by disdain for more supernatural perspectives, spiritual aspects of mental health are now receiving scientific examination. The importance of cultural competence for mental health professionals is now a given and spiritual competence is an essential element in cultural competence.

Discussion questions

1.   What culture(s) did you grow up with in your family?

2.   What culture(s) influence(s) you now? Why?

3.   How does the concept of intersectionality apply to you?

4.   How do your cultural context and identity limit your understanding of people from other cultures?

Exercise

Over two-thirds of today's refugees (68%) come from one of the following countries (Reid, 2021):

- Syria
- Venezuela
- Afghanistan
- South Sudan
- Myanmar (Rohingya)

Pick a culture from this list with which you are not familiar and research it online. Give a description of this culture and identify the cultural factors to which you would need to be especially sensitive in working with a refugee. Use the World Culture Encyclopedia listed below.

Resources

Religious/Spiritually Integrated Practice Assessment Scale: https://hollyoxhandler. com/wp-content/uploads/2020/04/Religious-Spirituality-Integrated-Practice-Assessment-Scale_v2_2016.pdf

The World Culture Encyclopedia contains a great deal of information about different cultures: https://www.everyculture.com/A-Bo/index.html

The Spiritual Competency Academy offers free online courses in spiritual competence: www.spiritualcompetencyacademy.com/

Chapter 3

What is Spirituality?

There are widely varying opinions about the meaning of the word spiritual and there is no single, agreed-upon definition. Defining spirituality is reminiscent of the Indian story about the men who were blind and who were trying to figure out what an elephant was by touching it. They were all touching the same creature, but each was touching a different part. To one an elephant was rough and scaly, to another it was small and snake-like, to another hard and horn-like, to a fourth it was wet and slimy, etc. An elephant is made up of many different shapes and textures. How they saw the elephant depended on what part of the elephant they touched. In what follows, we will discuss some of the ways in which the concept of spirituality has been used.

Emmons & Paloutzian (2003) observe that the noun "spirit" and the adjective "spiritual" are being used to refer to an ever-increasing range of experiences rather than being reserved for those occasions of use that specifically imply the existence of non-material forces or persons. They do not define spirituality in general but do define three specific types of spirituality: **Religious spirituality** is spirituality that is related to particular religious beliefs while **natural spirituality** involves the individual's relationship to and reverence toward the natural world. **Humanistic spirituality** considers spirituality as an aspect of human experience rather than a manifestation of the divine.

Senreich (2013) has proposed a definition that includes the entire spectrum of experience mentioned above:

> Spirituality refers to a human being's relationship (cognitive, emotional, and intuitive) to what is unknowable about existence, and how a person

integrates that relationship into a perspective about the universe, the world, others, self, moral values, and one's sense of meaning (p. 553).

Dudley (2016) gives a different definition:

Spirituality refers to a universal and fundamental human quality involving the search for a sense of meaning, purpose, morality, well-being, and profundity in relationships with ourselves, others, and ultimate reality.

Like Emmons & Paloutzian, Saunders *et al.* (2010) see the concept of spirituality as inclusive of religion and as encompassing both religious and non-religious strivings. These authors view religion as a narrower concept, applying specifically to systems of beliefs and practices that are formally defined by a religious organization.

In this book, "spiritual" will be used as the more inclusive term, with "religion" denoting the officially sanctioned beliefs and practices of various organized faith groups.

The word spirit also can have many different meanings, but for our purposes, spirit is considered to be the non-physical part of ourselves. Merriam-Webster defines it as "the immaterial intelligent or sentient part of a person". The word traces back to the Latin word spiritus, which means "breath". Breathing, of course, is what keeps us alive, and is a key element in many spiritual and religious traditions and practices. Spirit includes not just awareness, but also thought, meaning, motivation, and intentionality. In secular terms, spirit is seen as strictly a function of the brain and, like consciousness, is not believed to exist apart from the brain (Edelman, 2004). In a spiritual or religious context, however, spirit often has a broader meaning, applying to the part of a person that connects, or can connect, to God, the Divine, the holy, or the transcendent and that lives on or is reborn after death. This belief is central to many religions. Religions will be discussed in the next chapter.

Some of the words and phrases that have been used in various definitions of spirituality are:

- Faith or beliefs
- Asking the big questions
- Moral and ethical values
- Disciplines or practices
- Character strengths or virtues

- The pursuit of higher meaning
- A transcendent experience
- Connection to the whole/diminishing of ego
- A brain-based cognitive, emotional, and/or somatic state

3.1 Faith or beliefs

While the word spirituality is often used to indicate religious faith or beliefs, the faith or beliefs need not be religious to be spiritual and spiritual individuals are not necessarily affiliated with a formal religion. Hill *et al.* (2001) have pointed out that the distinction between religion and spirituality is a relatively new one, necessitated by the rise of secularism and increased disenchantment with religion in the U.S. and Great Britain during the latter half of the 20th century. This development coincided with a number of Eastern and Middle Eastern diasporas resulting from social and political conditions. These diasporas brought new spiritual disciplines and practices to the West ("New Age" spirituality). The word spirituality began to be used widely in the 1960s and 1970s to distinguish personal experiences of the transcendent from experiences occurring in a religious context.

It is interesting that many contemporary Anglo-European definitions of spirituality tend to make a point of distinguishing between spirituality and religion. This is not true in some other countries. For example, much of the Iranian literature observes that in this predominantly Islamic country, spirituality is generally conceived of as closeness to Allah and is not distinguished from religion (Ghorbani *et al.*, 2014; Marzband *et al.*, 2016; Memaryan *et al.*, 2016). Hindus, on the other hand, are more likely to consider all religions (and atheism) as potentially spiritual (Young & Sarin, 2014).

Hodge (2015, p. 11) has depicted the relationship between spirituality and religion in the form of a Venn diagram in which there is a large area of overlap between spirituality and religion. A similar diagram appears below with the addition of data from the Pew Research Center, which has conducted a U.S. survey asking people whether they are religious and whether they are spiritual (2017a). The percentages of respondents in the survey falling into each category have been entered into Figure 3.1. Almost half said they were both spiritual and religious while slightly more than a quarter said they were spiritual but not religious (often abbreviated in the social media as "SBNR"). 6% said they were religious but not spiritual, while 18% said they were neither spiritual nor religious.

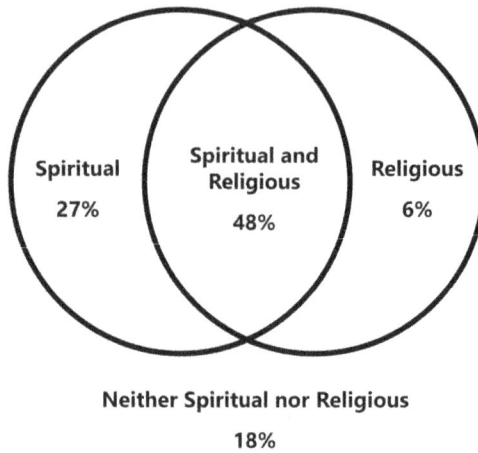

Figure 3.1.   Religion and spirituality.

There are differences among religious and cultural groups in the U.S., however. For example, U.S. Christians (62%) are somewhat more likely than U.S. Muslims (50%) to say they are both religious and spiritual (Pew Research Center, 2017b). Muslim immigrants to the U.S. are considerably less likely than those born in the U.S. to consider themselves either spiritual or religious. This may reflect immigrants' negative experiences with authoritarian Islam in their countries of origin, as well as the fact that the distinction between religion and spirituality is less commonly made in Islamic countries. There are also differences among countries in how religious or spiritual people report themselves as being. Another Pew survey (2018) of people in 15 Western European countries found that, in contrast to the U.S., only 24% identified themselves as "spiritual and religious" while 53% considered themselves neither religious nor spiritual. 11% said they were spiritual but not religious.

A belief in God is not necessary for one to consider oneself either religious or spiritual. As we shall see in the next chapter, not all religions assume the existence of a Divinity, but even if they did, spirituality does not necessarily imply a belief in a God or gods. The term **secular spirituality** is often used to characterize those who are spiritual but not religious. Fuller (2017) has identified eight features of secular spirituality:

1. Eclecticism
2. Self-growth

3. Relevance to life
4. Self-direction
5. Openness to wonder
6. Authenticity beyond churches
7. Metaphysical[1] explanations
8. Communal and ecological morality

As one might expect, the vast majority of U.S. atheists say religion is "not too" or "not at all" important in their lives (93%) and that they seldom or never pray (97%) (Pew Research Center, 2019). At the same time, many do not see a contradiction between atheism and pondering their place in the world. In fact, about a third of the American atheists studied say they think about the meaning and purpose of life at least weekly (35%) and the atheists are more likely than U.S. Christians to say they often feel a sense of wonder about the universe (54% vs. 45%). Throughout history, humans in all cultures, regardless of whether they believe in any divine power, have shown such an appreciation for the sacred or holy in their experience of their physical environment by designating certain locations or moments as special or other-worldly. Eugene Gendlin, the author of the book *Focusing* (1982), defines spirituality as "a subtle, bodily feeling with vague meanings that brings new, clearer meanings involving a transcendent growth process". The words "holy" and "sacred" are synonyms and have many meanings. They can refer to something related to a deity, but they can also mean any of the following:

• Something that is dedicated or set apart for a particular purpose
• Something that is worthy of spiritual respect or devotion
• Something that inspires awe or reverence
• Something of great value

One term for locations perceived as sacred or holy is "**thin places**". According to the ancient Celts, a thin place is a place where the veil between the physical dimension and the spiritual dimension is lifted. These can be

---

[1] Metaphysics is a discipline in philosophy that is concerned with the nature of reality and being.

sacred, mystical, or natural places but they may also be occasions, times or dates, or experiences. A thin place is a place that is numinous or filled with a supernatural presence. Some examples of sites considered by many to be thin places are:

- Bear Mountain, in Bear Butte State Park, sacred to the Lakota and Cheyenne Indians
- Mecca, in Saudi Arabia, site of the holy Kaaba, a small stone building containing a sacred black stone
- Glastonbury, in England, a sacred site for many spiritual traditions since 5000 BCE
- Bodh Gaya, in India, the site of Buddha's enlightenment
- St. Peter's Basilica, Rome, Italy
- Sedona, Arizona, considered by many to be a center of healing energy

Another relevant phrase is "**holy ground**". This expression originates in the Hebrew Scriptures. In the Book of Exodus, before the Holy One gives Moses the Ten Commandments, he tells him: "Do not approach here. Take off your sandals, for the place on which you are standing is holy ground." In this sense, holy ground is not a physical place but a spiritual place.

3.2 Moral or ethical behavior

Some believe that moral or ethical behavior is an element in spirituality (James, 1890, 1902; Walker, 2003). Humanistic spirituality often emphasizes moral and ethical conduct. Ethical Culture Societies, for example, are humanistic spiritual organizations that do not take a position on the existence of a God or higher power but emphasize the importance of moral or ethical behavior. Greg Epstein, a Humanist Rabbi Chaplain at Harvard University, is the president of the university's corps of over 40 chaplains from more than 20 different religions, and has written a book titled *Good Without God* (2009). In it he presents a secular perspective on morality and ethics. Research has by and large failed to demonstrate a connection between spirituality and moral or ethical behavior, however. Still, many people believe there is a connection. The Pew Research Center (2020a) has studied attitudes about this issue in 34 countries and found that, on average, 45% of those surveyed responded that a belief in God was necessary for a person to be moral and have good values. There were substantial differences among countries in this belief, however. Countries in which 80% or more of those surveyed felt a belief in God was necessary in order to be moral and have good values were: Indonesia (96%), Philippines (96%), Kenya (95%), Nigeria (93%), South Africa (84%), Brazil (84%), and Tunisia (84%). There were only three countries in which 80% or more of those surveyed felt a belief in God was not necessary: Sweden (90%), France (84%), and the Czech Republic (80%). The other countries studied ranged between these two extremes.

3.3 Disciplines or practices

A spiritual discipline or practice is a behavior performed or attitude cultivated for the purpose of spiritual growth or development. People who engage in spiritual practices are often considered to be spiritual people. Most common spiritual disciplines or practices were developed in the context of a religion, and many are shared among different religious traditions. It is not necessary to believe in a religion or belong to a religious group to engage in a spiritual practice, however. Some of the most widely shared are:

- **Meditation** — Maintaining focus on a particular object of attention regardless of distractions.
- **Movement** — The practice of certain movements to improve mind-body-spirit wholeness and health.
- **Prayer** — Asking for help, guidance, or blessing, whether or not the request is addressed to a deity.
- **Fasting** — Refraining from eating for a specified period.
- **Silence** — Refraining from speaking for a specified period.
- **Gratitude** — Affirming the positives in life and those who are responsible for them.
- **Solitude and/or silence** — Spending time alone and/or silent.
- **Forgiveness** — Letting go of resentment.
- **Generosity** — Giving freely and frequently to others.
- **Service** — Performing acts that are helpful to others.
- **Hope** — A feeling of trust that all will be well.
- **Agape** — Selfless or unconditional love, compassion.

It may seem strange to label such emotions as gratitude, forgiveness, service, or love as practices, but there is a reason for it. To practice something means to do it repeatedly to become better at it and make it automatic. Gratitude, forgiveness, hope, and love are acts we must perform repeatedly, whether we feel like it or not, if we want them to become automatic feelings and behaviors.

3.4 Character strengths/virtues

Some definitions of spirituality focus on character traits that are promoted by spiritual practices. Psychologists in the relatively new area of positive psychology have been interested in how character strength or virtues fostered by spiritual traditions and practices promote psychological well-being (e.g., Kim-Prieto, 2014a; Littman-Ovadia & David, 2020). Niemiec *et al.* (2020) point out that just as spirituality can foster character strengths, character strengths can enhance and deepen spiritual practices.

Peterson & Seligman (2004) have classified spiritual strengths deemed essential for the "good life" in the texts of seven major religious traditions — Confucianism, Taoism, Buddhism, Hinduism, ancient Greek, Judeo-Christianity, and Islam. They have identified six categories of virtue (in bold type below), consisting of 26 measurable character strengths (italicized below):

1. **Wisdom and Knowledge:** *creativity, curiosity, open-mindedness, love of learning, perspective, innovation*
2. **Courage:** *bravery, persistence, integrity, vitality, zest*
3. **Humanity:** *love, kindness, social intelligence*
4. **Justice:** *citizenship, fairness, leadership*
5. **Temperance:** *forgiveness and mercy, humility, prudence, self-control*
6. **Transcendence:** *appreciation of beauty and excellence, gratitude, hope, humor, spirituality*

Berry, Worthington, & O'Connor (2003) identified two major dimensions of character strength: **warmth-based virtues** such as empathy, sympathy, compassion, forgiveness, humility, and love, and **conscientiousness-based virtues** such as responsibility, accountability, justice, and self-control.

3.5 A search for higher meaning

To some, spirituality involves the search for some larger context or framework within which their life has meaning beyond day-to-day events. Viktor Frankel was a neurologist and psychiatrist who developed a school of psychotherapy that he called **logotherapy**. It was based on the premise that the attempt to find meaning in life was the primary motivation for humans. The goal of logotherapy was to help patients find personal meaning in their lives. Frankl was a key thinker in shaping the Existentialist movement and also the advocate of many concepts that later became integral to cognitive-behavioral psychotherapy. What is it like to find meaning in one's life? Essentially, this has to do with the story we tell ourselves about the purpose of our life and its connection to something larger than ourselves. In the Western world, perhaps as a result of what Max Weber called the "Protestant Ethic", great value is placed on productivity and material success. In many Asian countries, the purpose of existence is to live in such a way as to become liberated from the cycle of birth and rebirth. Existential theologians view spirituality as a concern with the big questions of existence or, in Tillich's words, matters of "**ultimate concern**" (2011). These are questions such as: What is the nature of the universe and what is my place in it? What is the purpose of life? Who am I, really? What is the meaning of my life? What happens when we die?

3.6 A transcendent experience

A transcendent experience involves connecting to a reality beyond the physical or material level. Hissan (2007) defines it from an Islamic perspective as an awareness of the Nafs (soul) during a higher level of consciousness, a state of perception and awareness of the cosmos. He notes that religious traditions have different names for such experiences: in Buddhism, it is "emptiness"; Jesus called it "Father"; Al-Halaj, a 10th-century Persian mystic, called it "Al-Haqq" ("truth", or "God"); and Sufis call it "the Beloved". William James' classic, *The Varieties of Religious Experience*, is a collection of his lectures that was first published in 1902 but has since been republished many times. In spite of its title, it is really concerned with spiritual rather than religious experience. James gives many examples of spiritual experiences. For the most part, they have the following characteristics:

- They feel real and significant.
- They reveal a reality beyond what we normally experience.
- They are temporary.
- They cannot be deliberately invoked.
- They are difficult, if not impossible, to describe in words.

Deborah Sokolove is a Professor Emerita at Wesley Theological Seminary and the former Director of the Henry Luce III Center for the Arts and Religion. She has observed that some researchers have categorized spiritual experiences according to the kinds of awareness they may involve (2021). These include:

- A patterning of events/synchronicity
- A spiritual presence, such as an angel or other spirit
- God or sense of being loved and/or at peace
- Prayer being answered
- A sacred presence in the natural world
- Oneness
- Evil, or an evil presence
- Ghosts, spirits, or other intimations of an afterlife

In 2008, Stark published the results of a survey that inquired about the religious and spiritual attitudes of U.S. adults. He asked about five "supernatural" experiences and found that more than half of the respondents reported one or more of the experiences listed in Table 3.1.

Stark found that people who had had one supernatural experience were likely to say they had had others. Slightly more than a quarter (27%) of those

Table 3.1. Experiences of the supernatural among the general public, U.S. (based on data from Stark, 2008).

Experience	%
I was protected from harm by a guardian angel	55
I felt called by God to do something	44
I heard the voice of God speaking to me	20
I witnessed a miraculous physical healing	23
I received a miraculous physical healing	16

surveyed said that they had had at least three of the experiences and almost one-fifth (18%) said they had had two. According to Stark, 45% of the respondents reported at least one experience that involved God. He also observed that women and African Americans were more likely than men and Anglo-Europeans to report multiple supernatural encounters. The term "**near-death experience**" was coined by Raymond Moody (1975) and since then has gained a great deal of popularity. It refers to an altered state of consciousness in an individual who has come very close to death or (technically) died but then been resuscitated. They are reported by about 17% of those who nearly die (Moore & Greyson, 2017). Koch (2020) lists the following frequently occurring elements of near-death experiences:

- Vision and hearing apart from the physical body
- Passing into or through a tunnel
- Encountering a mystical light
- Intense and generally positive emotions
- A review of part or all of their previous life
- Encountering deceased loved ones
- A choice to return to life

3.7 Connection to the whole/diminishing of ego

One feature of many transcendent experiences deserves its own section here. That is the sense of oneness and the loss of ego. Van Lente & Hogan (2020) studied the statements of experienced meditators from a variety of traditions about how they experienced "oneness" in their mediations and their daily lives. These were the most common responses:

- A recognition that suffering is part of oneness.
- A sense of no longer searching.
- A sense of trust in inner guidance.
- A sense of "being in eternal nowness".
- A sense of seeing that our nature is kindness.
- An awareness that all of one's actions have an effect on the universe.
- A sense of accessing one's true essence.

  "**Ego dissolution**" and "**ego death**" are phrases that are sometimes used to describe what happens during such experiences.

3.8 Spirituality as a brain-based cognitive, emotional, and/or somatic state

MacDonald *et al.* (2015) suggest a science-based approach to defining spirituality that emphasizes its experiential nature with certain characteristic neurophysiological, cognitive, characterological, and behavioral features. There has already been considerable research confirming that there are neurobiological correlates of transcendent experiences (Sayadmansour, 2014; Grafman *et al.*, 2020; Newberg, 2021). These brain states can exist with or without a belief in a deity or divine presence. This specialized field of study is known as "**neurotheology**" or "**spiritual neuroscience**". Researchers (Ferguson *et al.*, 2021) have found a relationship between reduced activity in the right parietal lobe of the brain and spirituality. Some psychoactive substances such as hallucinogens have been used in religious ceremonies and psychological research to induce transcendent states. Research has revealed a common core of experiences across cultures, religions, and degrees of religiosity regardless of whether transcendent experiences occur naturally or as a result of ingesting a substance (Newberg, 2021). Mihalyi Csiksentmihalyi (2008) has identified a state he calls "**flow**". Flow has many of the elements sometimes found in a transcendent experience, including intense engagement, positive feelings, loss of self-consciousness, and a changed perception of time. Interestingly, the neurological correlates of the state of flow include a suppression in the functioning of the frontal lobe, which is responsible for critical thinking and analysis, and an increased functioning of the part of the brain called the basal ganglia, which is responsible for the performance of well-practiced skills that require little conscious thought (Dietrich, 2004). This may be why the practice of martial arts and other movement-related systems are often used as meditation tools.

Porges' (2011) polyvagal theory is a relatively new perspective that offers a neurological explanation for transcendent states of connection and oneness. The theory has produced many useful tools for clinicians, though it does not, as yet, have enough research support to be widely accepted by the neuroscience community. The theory focuses on the ventral vagal aspect of the parasympathetic nervous system. The ventral vagal system responds to perceptions of external and internal safety and produces feelings of wellbeing, connection and social engagement. It also is responsible for a spiritual sense of wholeness and oneness with all that is.

In conclusion, a number of definitions and concepts have been presented in this chapter. Some, such as "spirituality" and "spirit", have no generally agreed-upon definition, so that one must be careful to define the terms when using them in a discussion. Many are defined differently depending on whether they are being used in a religious, spiritual, or secular context. A distinction was made between religious, natural, and humanistic spirituality. Religions generally have a spiritual component, but one need not be religious or embrace one specific religion to be spiritual. Attitudes, behaviors, or experiences considered by some to be spiritual include beliefs, values, practices, virtues, pursuit of higher meaning, transcendence, unity, and ego loss. In addition, in recent years more is being learned about neurological processes underlying various kinds of spiritual experiences. As used in this book, spirituality is inclusive of religion. Spirituality denotes a person's thoughts, feelings, and behaviors related to "concern about, a search for, or a striving for understanding and relatedness to the transcendent" (Hill *et al.*, 2001). Thus, spirituality encompasses both religious and non-religious strivings. The concept of religion is narrower, as it refers to a particular system of beliefs and behaviors that is formally sanctioned by an external entity, such as a church body (Hill *et al.*, 2001). For many people, spiritual thoughts, feelings, and behaviors are related to an identifiable religion, but they can be pursued outside the auspices of any religion.

Discussion questions

1. This chapter presents many different meanings for the word spirituality. Can you think of a meaning that is not mentioned in this chapter? If so, what is it?

2. People are often reluctant to speak openly about their spiritual experiences. Why do you think this is?

3. What does spirituality mean to you?

4. How important is spirituality in your life?

5. Have you ever had a "transcendent experience"? What was it like?

Exercise

Ask five people:

1. Whether they consider themselves to be a spiritual person and why (or why not).
2. Whether they consider themselves as religious and why (or why not).

Then write one page or less explaining your results and what you learned from them.

Resources

Spirituality and Practice is a multifaith and interspiritual website devoted to resources for spiritual journeys: https://www.spiritualityandpractice.com/about/about-sp

Institute for Spiritual and Health virtual resources: https://www.spiritualityandhealth.org/resources

Chapter 4

Religions

The Pew Research Center, based on global census figures, estimates that, worldwide, more than eight in ten people identify with a religious group (2012). Figures vary among and within countries, however. Based on telephone interviews with a random sample of 50,000 Americans (Cox & Jones, 2017), it is reported that there has been a generational shift in religious affiliation in the U.S. Only 12% of Americans 65 and over identify as unaffiliated compared to 38% of those between 18 and 29 years old. Among those between 30 and 49, 26% say they are unaffiliated while the figure for those between 50 and 64 is 18%.

Religion is a concept that is as difficult to define as spirituality and there is much disagreement among theologians as to what constitutes a religion. The Merriam-Webster dictionary includes the following definitions of religion:

- The service and worship of God or the supernatural.
- Commitment or devotion to religious faith or observance.
- A personal set or institutionalized system of religious[1] attitudes, beliefs, and practices.

Critics have argued that there is an inherent Judeo-Christian and Western bias in this kind of definition of religion (e.g., Smith, 1991; Dubuisson, 2007; Fitzgerald, 2007; Nye, 2018). Most definitions include

---

[1] Merriam-Webster defines the word "religious" in a circular fashion as: "believing in God or gods and following the practices of a religion".

such concepts as a worship of a deity, an organized body of believers, a shared system of beliefs, and/or rules and practices. While most sociologists and anthropologists consider religion to be a cultural universal, the religions of many cultures over time have lacked one or more of these elements. Fitzgerald notes that the concept of religion itself is far from universal and most likely did not even emerge until the 4th century AD, when Christianity was invoked by the Roman emperor Constantine to strengthen his power as he sought to expand the Roman Empire. Colonialism seems to have been a major factor in spreading the concept of religion to cultural groups that did not originally conceptualize their spiritual lives in these terms (Day, 2020; Fitzgerald, 2007; Goulet, 2011; Nye, 2018). At the extreme, it has also been argued that the concept of religion is one created by theologians and other academics rather than a reflection of reality. Smith (1991), the influential scholar who popularized this idea, states that religion, far from being a cultural universal, is "solely the creation of the scholar's study and has no independent existence apart from the academy".

One feature of most definitions of religion is that they imply a distinction between the religious and the secular, with the term secular referring to anything that is not explicitly religious. But as we shall soon see, there are many cultures that make no distinction between the religious and the secular, notably indigenous religions and their contemporary offshoots. Houtman & Meyer (2013) attribute this narrow focus of standard definitions of religion to the Western, and specifically Protestant, belief that the material and the spiritual are mutually exclusive. The imposition of this distinction on other cultures has been one result of colonialization. Nelson (2009) distinguishes between definitions of religion that focus on transcendence, or spiritual experiences beyond the physical dimension of reality, and those that focus on immanence, or activities in the material dimension of existence. He notes that some religions focus on transcendence while others focus on immanence but points out that the major world religions focus on both. Pesut *et al.* (2008) argue against a distinction frequently made between spirituality and religion. In this distinction, spirituality is viewed as an individual characteristic or experience while religion is seen as a group function with institutionalized beliefs and rituals. In fact, as discussed in the previous chapter, there is tremendous overlap between spirituality and religion. Religions are spiritual in nature and spirituality often finds its expression in organized religions. Individuals can be spiritual but not religious, religious but not spiritual, both, or neither. In fact, Verghese (2008) defines religion as "institutionalized spirituality". This definition, too, can be disputed since there are organizations that are spiritual but not explicitly religious (i.e., mindfulness meditation or ethical humanist groups and societies). For the purposes of this book, religion will be treated as a sub-category of spirituality, since all religions have some kind of a spiritual component while not all spiritual orientations have a religious component.

In this chapter, religious traditions are grouped into categories based on their commonalities. There is a certain arbitrariness to these categories because the groupings depend on which commonalities we choose to emphasize and which we choose to ignore. These groups could easily have been entirely different if we had chosen differently. Some of the religions could have been placed in more than one category. Furthermore, each tradition is extremely diverse within itself and varies considerably from one geographic area to another and from one individual to another. It is important to remember not to rely on stereotypes in attempting to understand a client's religious orientation. The Pew Research Center conducts a number of ongoing international studies of religious life. Based on a worldwide study of censuses, surveys, and population records, it has produced Figure 4.1 depicting the world's largest religious groups (2012).

4.1 Abrahamic religions

Judaism, Christianity, and Islam have common roots and are often called the Abrahamic religions because they are believed to have originated with the scriptural figure of Abraham either directly or through one or the other of his two sons (Figure 4.2). The Pew Research Center (2012) estimates that approximately 55% of the world's population belongs to one of the Abrahamic traditions.

In discussing the Abrahamic religions, it is important to remember that they were influenced by a mixture of other faith traditions that were present in the Middle East before, during, and after the supposed time of Abraham. The most influential earlier tradition was probably Zoroastrianism. One of

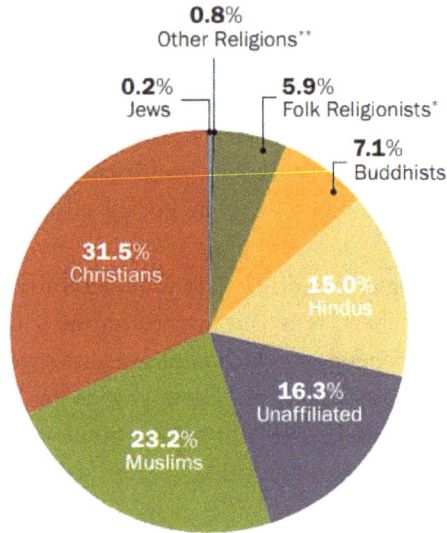

Size of Major Religious Groups, 2010

Percentage of the global population

0.8% Other Religions**
0.2% Jews
5.9% Folk Religionists*
7.1% Buddhists
31.5% Christians
15.0% Hindus
16.3% Unaffiliated
23.2% Muslims

*Includes followers of African traditional religions, Chinese folk religions, Native American religions and Australian aboriginal religions.

**Includes Baha'i's, Jains, Sikhs, Shintoists, Taoists, followers of Tenrikyo, Wiccans, Zoroastrians and many other faiths.

Percentages may not add to 100 due to rounding.

Figure 4.1.   Major religions of the world (Pew Research Center, 2012).

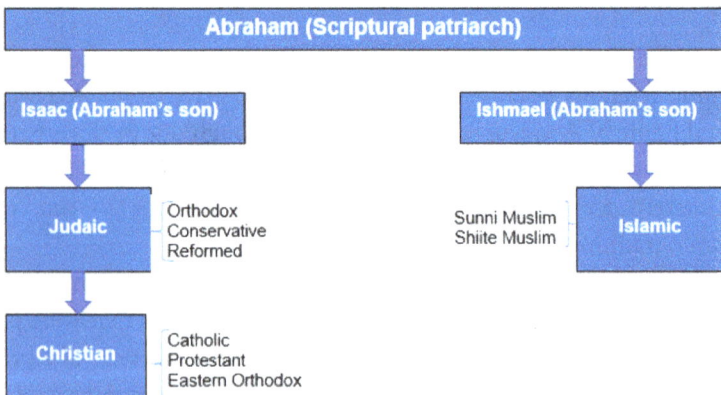

Abraham (Scriptural patriarch)

Isaac (Abraham's son)

Ishmael (Abraham's son)

Judaic — Orthodox / Conservative / Reformed

Sunni Muslim / Shiite Muslim — Islamic

Christian — Catholic / Protestant / Eastern Orthodox

Figure 4.2.   The Abrahamic religions and their major branches.

the oldest, still-practiced religions, its central theme is the cosmic struggle between good and evil. It is a theistic religion, meaning that it is characterized by a belief in a god, or gods. There are numerous traditions branching out from every level of Figure 4.2. For example, Reconstructionist Judaism is a denomination of Judaism that is nontheistic and rejects many Jewish beliefs, including the belief that Jews are the chosen people. The Anglo-Catholics in the U.S. and the United Kingdom and the Old Catholics in Europe are sects (Table 4.1) that separated from the Catholic Church but do not consider themselves Protestant.

Table 4.1.   Some definitions of words used in religion.

Religious tradition	Beliefs, customs, practices, and behaviors that define a religion.
Orthodox	Adhering to the original doctrine and practices of a religion.
Fundamentalism	Strict literalism in the interpretation of orthodox beliefs and writings, along with a desire to return to an earlier ideal and a rejection of out-groups. Can result in political conflict (e.g., Buddhist fundamentalist persecution of Muslim Rohingya in Myanmar; Muslim persecution of religious minorities in Pakistan; Christian terrorists attacks on Jews in the U.S.).
Denomination	A recognized, autonomous, widely accepted branch of a religion that shares its name, tradition, and identity (i.e., Sunni/Muslim; Presbyterian/Christian; Shaktism/Hindu; Reformed/Judaism).
Sect	An offshoot or subgroup of a religion that deviates in some way from the original doctrine and practices of the religion. It is smaller than a denomination and has a shorter history but may eventually become a denomination (for example, Mormonism began as a sect but is now a Christian denomination). Sects may be viewed as heretical by the original religion.
Heresy	A heresy is a doctrine or belief system rejected as false by a religious authority and labeled heretical.
Interfaith	Interaction or cooperation among differing religions or faith organizations.
Ecumenical	Interaction or cooperation among differing Christian denominations.
Proselytize	To convert or attempt to convert someone to one's own religion.
Conversion	Deciding to adopt a religion or changing one's belief from one religion to another.
Religiosity	The strength of a person's religious beliefs.

Some Rastafarians, adherents of a Jamaican religion with Judeo-Christian roots, consider themselves Christian and some do not. The Sufi religion, a mystical version of Islam, is considered by some to be a branch of Islam but by most Sufis to transcend religious categories. The Sufi tradition is rejected by fundamentalist Muslims who do not consider it a true Islamic religion. Though there are many Abrahamic religions, denominations, and sects, there are significant commonalities among most of them. Some of their shared beliefs are shown in Table 4.2.

Another commonality among these religions, probably attributable to their Zoroastrian roots, is the belief in good and evil as opposing forces. This contrasts with some Eastern bodies of belief, such as Taoism, which see good and evil (light and dark) as complementary parts of the same whole. In comparing the Abrahamic traditions, it is interesting to note that Christian and Muslim beliefs have more in common with each other than either one has with Judaism, even though all three have common origins. Both Islam and Christianity hold that Jesus was born of the Virgin Mary, that Jesus is God's prophet and messenger, and that God revealed the Gospel through Jesus. Both belief systems include an afterlife while Judaism is not clear on this. Islam differs from the other traditions in believing that Muhammed was the final prophet and messenger of God and that the name of the Divine Being is Allah. Christianity is alone in believing in a three-part divinity (Creator/Christ/Holy Spirit), in original sin, and in Christ as a Savior who died to redeem humans from their sins (though Islam acknowledges Jesus as a prophet).

It is important to remember that there is a great deal of variation among individuals and within specific faith organizations that consider themselves a part of the Abrahamic tradition in the extent to which they embrace the

Table 4.2.   Shared beliefs of the Abrahamic religions.

- Devotion and surrender to a single God
- Belief that God is merciful and forgiving
- The Divine Being revealed the Torah (Hebrew Bible) through Moses
- The Divine Being revealed the Psalms through David
- Prayer is necessary in one's relationship to the Divine Being
- Humans must follow certain laws
- Humans must abide by certain values and ethical principles
- Humans will be held accountable on a judgment day

Abrahamic beliefs described above and to which they honor other beliefs not described above. For example, Messianic[2] Judaic groups such as Jews for Jesus combine traditional elements of Judaism with elements of Christianity that are not usually considered a part of Judaism. Jehovah's Witnesses are considered Christian, but they do not believe in an afterlife or in a triune Deity. The Bahai faith is an Abrahamic religion because it is an offshoot of Shia Islam but many of its beliefs differ from those of other Islamic groups, which sometimes results in the persecution of its members by Muslim fundamentalists. Still, Table 4.2 is helpful for appreciating the numerous commonalities among the three mainstream Abrahamic traditions. The words used in the Abrahamic religions to describe non-believers (atheist and agnostic) reflect the monotheistic (Figure 4.3) orientation of that tradition.

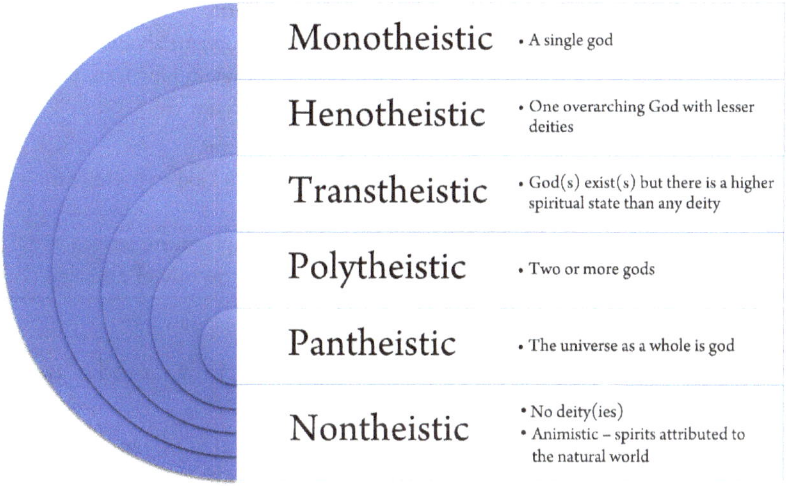

Monotheistic	• A single god
Henotheistic	• One overarching God with lesser deities
Transtheistic	• God(s) exist(s) but there is a higher spiritual state than any deity
Polytheistic	• Two or more gods
Pantheistic	• The universe as a whole is god
Nontheistic	• No deity(ies) • Animistic – spirits attributed to the natural world

Figure 4.3. Types of theism.

4.2 Dharmic Eastern religions

Hinduism, Buddhism, Sikhism and Jainism are often referred to as Eastern or Dharmic religions (Table 4.3). Hinduism originated in India. Buddhism began in India and spread to China, Japan, and Southeast Asia, where it took

---

[2] The word messianic refers to a belief that a divine being has appeared or will appear and will save believers or the world.

Table 4.3.   Major Dharmic Eastern religions.

Religion	Deities	Major Beliefs
Hinduism	Henotheistic Main gods are Brahma, Vishnu, and Shiva	• Reincarnation/Karma • Caste system • Goal is union with Brahma and release from cycle of rebirth (moksha)
Buddhism	Nontheistic/Transtheistic Archetypal deities more important in some lineages than others	• Reincarnation/Karma • Goal is liberation from cycle of rebirth and attainment of enlightenment, nirvana, or egolessness • Eightfold Path to enlightenment • Four Noble Truths (suffering, its cause, ending suffering, path to ending suffering)
Jainism	Transtheistic	• Reincarnation/Karma • Goal is heaven (Supreme abode) • Non-violence, religious pluralism, non-attachment, asceticism
Sikhism	Monotheistic	• Reincarnation/Karma • Goal is union with God and release from cycle of rebirth • Prayer, honest employment, generosity • Gender equality, rejection of caste and class

on different forms. Sikhism originated in South Asia, in what today are India and Pakistan. Jainism began in India.

Currently these religions are found in many parts of the world. One thing they have in common is a belief in reincarnation and Karma. The ultimate goal of life is to achieve liberation from the cycle of birth, death, and reincarnation by living a virtuous life. Karma is the sum of good and bad acts in a person's present or past lives which determines their circumstances in subsequent rebirths. The Four Noble Truths are:

1. Life is suffering.
2. The cause of suffering is craving.
3. The end of suffering comes with an end to craving.
4. There is a path which leads one away from craving and suffering.

The path alluded to in the fourth truth is The Eightfold Path which serves as both a guide on the road to non-attachment and the road itself. The precepts both inform a traveler on how to proceed and provide the way through spiritual discipline. The eight precepts are:

1. Right View
2. Right Intention
3. Right Speech
4. Right Action
5. Right Livelihood
6. Right Effort
7. Right Mindfulness
8. Right Concentration

The greater the number of good acts, the more positive the karma, and the more quickly the person will be released from the cycle of reincarnation and achieve union with the Divine.

Sikhism is a syncretic religion that combines Hinduism and Islam. The term **syncretism** refers to the incorporation into a religion of beliefs from a different, unrelated tradition. In a sense, all except the very earliest religions are syncretic because they have all been influenced by religions that came before them. A common cause of syncretism is the imposition of the religion of a dominant culture on an indigenous society due to conquest, colonization, or enslavement. An example of syncretism is the observation of the Days of the Dead in Mexico. The "Dia de los Muertos" celebrations originally reflect ancient indigenous burial customs and a belief that the spirits of the dead come alive at this time to visit their relatives in cemeteries. These beliefs have been incorporated into Catholic celebrations of All Saints' Day and All Souls' Day which were imposed on the indigenous people of Mexico by Spanish conquerors. Figure 4.4 shows a temporary Day of the Dead altar constructed in front of the permanent altar of a Catholic Church in Mexico.

The Pew Research Center (2012) reports that 15% of the world's population is affiliated with Hinduism and 7.1% with Buddhism. The other Dharmic religions are not tabulated separately but are grouped with "other religions" (0.8% of the world's population).

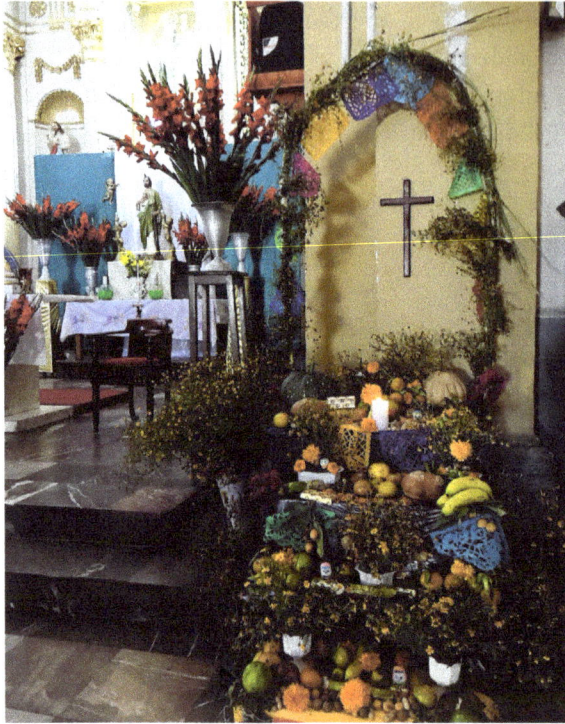

Figure 4.4. A Day of the Dead altar in a Catholic church in Mexico.

Table 4.4. Major nontheistic Eastern religions/philosophies.

Religion	Deities	Major Beliefs
Confucianism	No deities	• Importance of correct social relationships • Filial piety • Five key relationships (ruler-subject, father-son, elder brother-younger brother, husband-wife, friend-friend)
Taoism (Daoism)	No deities	• Tao is the force that governs everything in the universe • Goal is attunement with the natural universe, or Tao • Good is anything that flows with the way of the Tao, evil is anything that blocks it

There are two major philosophies of Asian origin that are often treated as religions, though they are nontheistic and concern themselves primarily with proper behavior (Table 4.4). They are Confucianism and Taoism (also called Daoism). Confucianism originated in China with the teachings of

Confucius in the 6th century BCE and is focused on the social order, stressing hierarchy and patriarchy. Over the centuries, Confucianism has spread to many Asian countries influenced by Chinese settlers or occupiers. Taoism also originated in China in the writings of Lao Tzu, a philosopher who wrote around the 5th century BCE. His main writing is known as the Tao Te Ching. Taoism stresses attunement with the natural universe. Neither tradition stresses reincarnation or an afterlife though both may include the commemoration or veneration of (male) ancestors.

"**Ancestor reverence**" is the appropriate term for what is commonly called "ancestor worship". Worship implies that the object of worship is seen as a deity, while reverence signifies only great admiration and respect. Ancestor reverence is common in many parts of Asia and occurs in other areas of the world as well. It is similar, in many respects, to the Catholic veneration of saints. Among those who practice ancestor reverence, it may be an obligation required by filial piety. In some variants, the spirits of deceased ancestors are believed to have the ability to intercede in earthly affairs on behalf of their descendants. When this is the case, families may create home altars dedicated to deceased ancestors. Sometimes offerings thought to be pleasing to the deceased such as flowers, food, or drinks are placed on the altars. Figure 4.5 shows a family altar in Mexico, created for the Days of the Dead celebration.

4.3 Animistic religions

Some religions are called animistic because they do not make a distinction between the material world and the spiritual world (Table 4.5). Instead, they see everything in nature, animate and inanimate, as imbued with spirit. Shintoism is the indigenous religion of Japan and, along with Buddhism, is one of Japan's two major religions. Indigenous religions are the religions of the original occupants of an area. They are typically animistic and therefore do not distinguish between the sacred and the secular. In many parts of the world indigenous religions have been wiped out by colonial forces that see them as a threat to their dominance or absorbed into the religions of the colonial powers. Neopagan religions, as described by White (2016), are "a collection of modern religious, spiritual, and magical traditions that are self-consciously inspired by the indigenous, pre-Judaic, pre-Christian, and pre-Islamic belief systems of Europe, North Africa, and the Near East". Wicca is

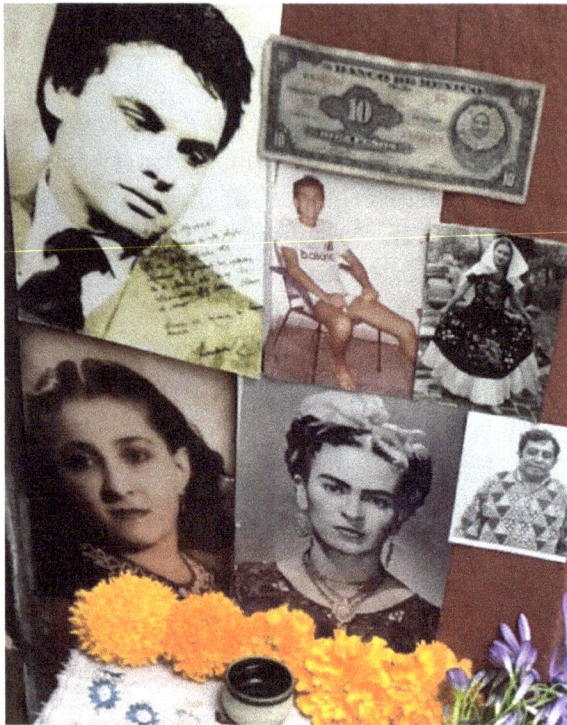

Figure 4.5.   An altar for Days of the Dead in Mexico.

Table 4.5.   Major animistic religions.

Religion	Deities	Major Beliefs
Indigenous	Animistic	All living and non-living beings have a spirit. Many have a concept of an afterlife, especially after domination by Western or Middle Eastern societies.
Shintoism	Animistic	All living and non-living things have a spirit. Ancestral spirits remain on earth, where they are worshipped by and protect their descendants.
Neopagan/ **Wicca**	Animistic/ Pantheistic	Modern religions inspired by indigenous religions. Diverse beliefs and practices.

the Neopagan religion that is most well known in the West. There is considerable diversity in the beliefs and practices of Wicca and other Neopagan groups, depending on which ancient or indigenous religions they aim to revive.

While all religions are influenced by the religions that came before them, the adoption of a culture's beliefs and practices by groups or individuals who are not native is viewed negatively by those who see it as another example of members of a dominant society exploiting a marginalized people (Pearson, 2002). Rouse (2014) points out how the idealization of American Indian spiritual practices is a form of "**cultural appropriation**". The expression refers to the out-of-context use of one or more elements of the culture of a (usually marginalized) group by another (usually dominant) group. Those who appropriate indigenous religious practices or sacred objects do not understand the worldview in which they are embedded and are not trained in their use. The separation of indigenous practices from the culture that shaped them and the guides who know how to use them can be harmful to outsiders who embrace these practices without proper guidance and disempowers indigenous teachers and authorities. In addition, the use of a society's sacred objects without understanding and honoring their intended meaning and purpose is often seen as a sacrilege.

4.4 Folk religions

Folk religions involve beliefs and practices that may have originated in an established religion but that have developed outside of the formal structure of that religion. They may be syncretic, including elements of earlier indigenous religions along with more recent (usually imposed) religious elements. Folk religions may be practiced alongside a formal religion but often involve deities or saints not recognized by that religion. Folk religion may include informally defined sacred objects, spaces, and places of worship. They also may include activities and procedures that are frowned on by local religious leaders, though such leaders often look the other way. Sinha (2007) describes some elements of "folk Hinduism" in Singapore:

> A pantheon of (non-Hindu) deities…spirit mediums and trance sessions…
> the importance of devotion, intuition, emotion and religious experience,
> the offerings of non-vegetarian items, alcohol and cigars to the deity, the
> absence of formalized, standardized and textually derived ritual procedures
> for approaching the deity, valuing rituals of self-mortification and other
> 'extreme' bodily rituals (p. 104).

Figure 4.6(a) shows a wooden statue of the Guatemalan folk saint, Maximón, probably derived from an ancient Mayan deity. Here, Maximón is

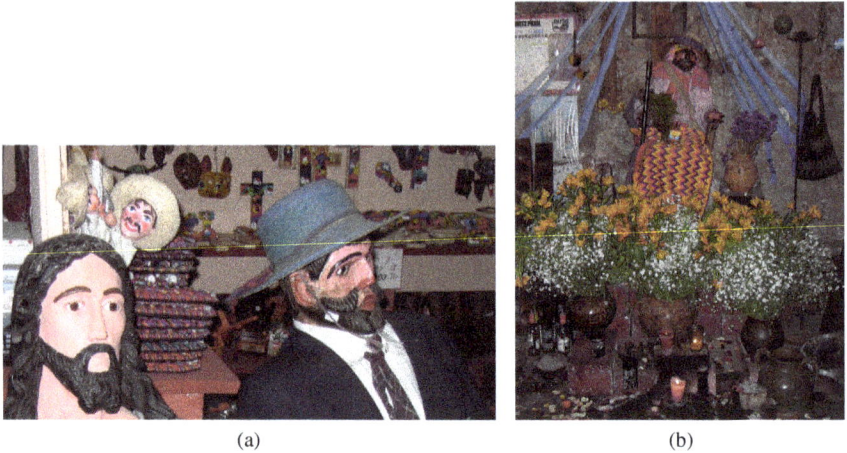

Figure 4.6.   (a) A statue of Maximón (right) next to a statue of Jesus in a souvenir shop. (b) Liquor and cigarette offerings to Maximón at an altar.

seated next to a statue of Jesus in an Antigua souvenir shop. Offerings to Maximón left at altars dedicated to him often include liquor or cigarettes because he is known to be a heavy drinker and smoker, as depicted in Figure 4.6(b). Prayers to Maximón are officially seen as taboo by the Catholic church and many of his followers believe that he answers prayers that a Catholic saint would refuse to answer because they are too corrupt. Nevertheless, statues or pictures of the Virgin Mary and other Catholic saints are often placed on his altars.

Another folk saint of the Americas is Santa Muerte ("Saint Death"), pictured in Figure 4.7. She is believed to be a syncretic version of a pre-Columbian Aztec death deity. Her petitioners, like those of Maximón, are condemned by Christian religious leaders but her followers are growing rapidly in Mexico, partly, but by no means entirely, due to her adoption as a patron saint by Mexican drug cartels. This has caused her to be labelled a "narcosaint", but she is also venerated by many of those on the other side of the drug war — police, soldiers, and prison guards (Kingsbury & Chesnut, 2020). Bromley (2016) notes that Santa Muerte is also especially popular among poor and marginal populations in Mexico.

4.5 Occult traditions

This category spans a tremendous variety of faiths and organizations, all of which embrace, to some degree, supernatural, mystical, or magical beliefs

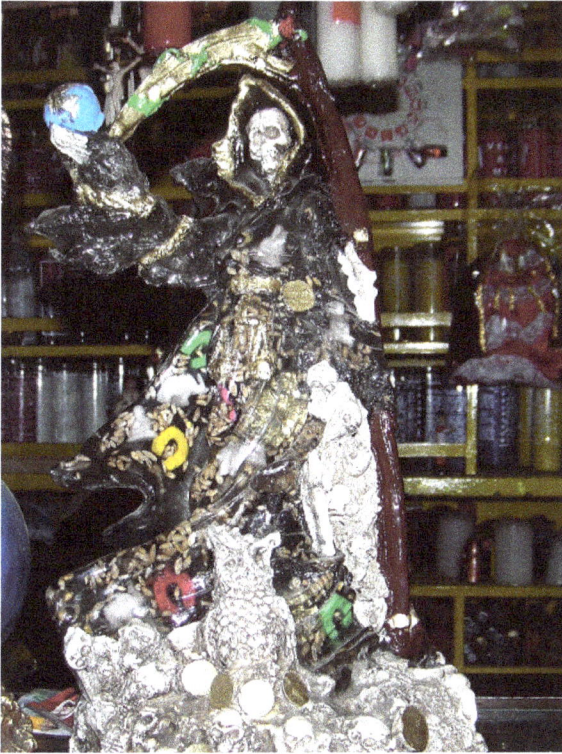

Figure 4.7.   A statue of Santa Muerte.

and practices (Table 4.6). Occult traditions fall outside the recognized domain of orthodox religions though they may have their own organizations and orthodoxies. Some occult religions are esoteric, meaning that they restrict their membership to a select few and may have stages leading to full membership. Some occult religious groups can be considered cults (see Section 4.6). Many are considered sacrilegious or dangerous by mainstream religions and have been vilified by orthodox believers and conspiracy theorists. For example, though the author of the Harry Potter series of children's books about a school for young wizards describes herself as Christian, both conservative Christian and Islamic writers have condemned the books (Abbot, 2007; Wilkinson, 2018). BBC News reported in 2019 that a group of Catholic priests in Poland included Harry Potter books in a collection of books they burned as sacrilegious. Doostdar (2019) points out that while Islam has a long tradition of occult writings and practices, the current revival

Table 4.6.   Some major occult traditions.

Tradition	Description
Spiritualism	A religious movement based on the belief that the spirits of the dead can communicate with the living.
Kabbalism	A Jewish esoteric mystical tradition.
Rosacrucianism	A worldwide brotherhood claiming to possess ancient knowledge about the metaphysical law governing the universe.
Taoist magic	A Taoist esoteric magical tradition.
Shamanism/ Neo- Shamanism	Originally referred to the practices of indigenous healers and visionaries who journeyed in a trance-like state to enlist the help of spirits. The term neo-Shamanism is a modern term that refers to any attempt to enter a trance-like state to contact the spirit world.
Voodoo	Caribbean syncretic traditions combining West African funerary customs* with Catholic saints, symbols, and practices.
Satanism	It is not really possible to offer a single definition of this tradition because it contains many very different large and small groups that call themselves Satanists. The most well-known group of Satanists is probably the Church of Satan, founded by Anton LaVey in 1966. Satanism is completely different from Wicca, neopaganism, or other occult traditions in that its beliefs, practices, theology, and moral values are deliberately antithetical to those of Christianity. Some Satanist traditions are simply anti-Christian while others actually worship Satan as a deity.

*Funerary customs are beliefs and practices used to remember and respect the dead.

of interest in the occult places many Iranians in conflict with Islamic religious orthodoxy.

Satanism, in particular, has been a topic that evokes fear and often triggers what have been called "**satanism scares**". One such famous scare was the McMartin preschool sexual abuse case in which bizarre allegations of satanic ritual sexual abuse resulted in charges being filed against a California day care center. The charges, made in 1983, were ultimately dismissed, but the investigation and trials lasted until 1990. Though the scare began in the U.S., it also spread to Canada, England, Australia, and other countries (Introvigne, 2000). More recently, in 2016, a rumor that a pizzeria in Washington, DC was a meeting place for satanic ritual child sexual abuse was spread widely through social media and resulted in threats, harassment, and attacks directed toward the pizzeria, its owners, and its staff.

4.6 Cults

The word "cult" is often loosely applied to any group of people that show an intense devotion to something or someone, for example: a cause, a popular figure or group, a movie, or a belief. When used in this way, it is not necessarily a pejorative term. Most cults are harmless and many eventually become denominations or complete religions. Mormonism, as already mentioned, began as a cult and became a denomination of Christianity. In fact, Christianity itself began as a cult.

Because cult is typically used as a derogatory term, many scholars now call cults "**new religions**" or "**new religious movements**" to avoid the negative implications of the word cult. These terms also lack a single, agreed-upon definition, and are applied to groups that differ widely in the degree to which they are controlling or exploitative.

New religious movements have always existed but their numbers began increasing markedly in the U.S. and elsewhere during the 1960s and 70s. While most of these groups were positive, or at least harmless, some dangerous cults did emerge with catastrophic consequences. In 1978, in Jonestown, Guyana, 918 members of a cult called the People's Temple drank poison at the command of their leader, an American named Jim Jones. During the 1990s, a cult named the Order of the Solar Temple was responsible for a number of mass suicides and murders in Canada, Switzerland, and France. Also during the 1990s, a Japanese cult, Aum Shinrikyō, released sarin, a poisonous gas, in the Tokyo subway system, killing 13 people and injuring 5,500. In 1997, 39 members of the Heaven's Gate cult in California committed suicide at the command of their leader. These and other developments during these decades engendered a "moral panic" and led to the development of what has been called the "**anti-cult movement**" in North America and, eventually, internationally. **Moral panic** is a widespread fear that some evil is taking over society (Jenkins, 1988). The concept was first introduced by Stanley Cohen in 1973 in his book, *Folk Devils and Moral Panic*. "**Folk devils**" are images of evil created and/or popularized by the media in narratives with the following characteristics:

- **Symbolization**: Portrayal of folk devil is oversimplified to make it easily recognizable.
- **Exaggeration**: Facts are distorted or fabricated to support a moral crusade.

- **Prediction**: Further immoral actions on the part of the folk devil are predicted.

Expert opinions are often used to support these narratives. Anti-cult activists, often family members of adults who had joined a cult or former cult members themselves, accused cults of "brainwashing" their members. Brainwashing is a term that developed during the Korean War to describe Chinese attempts to change the political values and beliefs of American prisoners of war using intensive and coercive techniques of indoctrination. The term **deprogramming** was coined in the 1970s to refer to attempts to reverse the effects of presumed cult brainwashing by convincing a person that their mind had been controlled by others and coercing them into adopting more conventional beliefs. Deprogramming was most often involuntary and could involve using some of the same intensive techniques as those used in brainwashing by the Chinese. The person to be deprogrammed was sometimes kidnapped and held hostage by a deprogrammer who was often paid exorbitant fees by relatives. Many experts spoke out against deprogramming, pointing out that the techniques used were unethical and a violation of civil rights. By the mid-1990s, courts began recognizing the illegality of many deprogramming techniques and the process died out, to be replaced by a process called "exit counseling". Exit counseling is voluntary — the person can leave at any time — and involves a focus on building a relationship and using it to change the person's beliefs.

Anti-cult activists often cite Robert Lifton, a psychiatrist who has written extensively on cults. Lifton argues that "mind control" is the central feature of a cult. Many of Lifton's writings deal with political cults such as Maoist groups in China during the Cultural Revolution, but he also writes about religious cults. Lifton acknowledges that some prefer the term "new religious movements" to the term cult and lists three criteria that distinguish cults from other groups and organizations (2019):

- Worship of a charismatic guru.
- The active pursuit of thought reform-like processes.
- Extensive exploitation (economic, sexual, or psychological) of followers by the guru and leading disciples.

There is no doubt that some new religious movements are dangerous. Groups such as the People's Temple, the Solar Temple, and Aum Shinrikyō have caused many innocent people to lose their lives. While most new religions are relatively small and many are short-lived, there are also large, international, new religious movements that many consider to be cults. Table 4.7 lists some

Table 4.7. Some international "new religious movements".

New Religious Movement	Description
Unification Church	This Church was founded in 1954 in Seoul, South Korea. Its members are sometimes called "Moonies" after their South Korean leader, Sun Myung Moon. The Church considers itself Christian and its teaching are based on the Bible but contain many new interpretations that are not accepted by Christian and Jewish religious leaders. It is involved in many business ventures and is a strong political force.
Church of Scientology	The Church of Scientology was founded in 1953 by L. Ron Hubbard and is based on his psychological theory called Dianetics. Its doctrines include a belief that humans are immortal spiritual beings who have lived previous extraterrestrial lives. Like Unification Church, the Church of Scientology is involved in numerous business ventures.
Eckankar	Eckankar, founded in 1965, is a group that has members in over 100 countries. A basic belief of Eckankar is that the soul can travel separately from the body and, in doing so, find its way back to God. Its practices include spiritual exercises designed to facilitate this journey.
International Society for Krishna Consciousness	Usually referred to as the Hare Krishna movement, this society was formed in 1966. Its core beliefs are based on the Hindu scriptures and the practice of Bhakti yoga, the cultivation of unconditional spiritual love toward a personal deity. One hallmark of this movement is the repetitive chanting of the "Hare Krishna" mantra.
Transcendental Meditation	A movement founded by Maharishi Mahesh Yogi in India in the mid-1950s. It is not clear whether this is an actual religious movement or simply a meditation technique. The technique involves the use of the silent repetition of a mantra given by a trained Transcendental Meditation teacher. The Transcendental organization is involved in many business ventures and charges fees for its training courses.
Rastafarianism	An Afrocentric religious movement that originated among poor and marginalized Afro-Jamaican communities in the 1930s in reaction to British colonialism. Haile Selassie, former Emperor of Ethiopia, is idealized and cannabis is regarded as a sacrament with beneficial properties. Members typically wear their hair in dreadlocks (twisted or rolled braids).

examples. Much anti-cult literature condemns the organizations listed in the table, as well as other similar, less well-known groups, accusing them of qualifying as cults according to Lifton's criteria. Others object to the moral panic-inducing position of anti-cult activists. Harrison (2016) sees the use of the term "cult" as simple prejudice against unorthodox religions. Though one can argue that cults deserve special attention because some are dangerous, Harrison argues that established religions have been responsible for far more bloodshed than cults. He believes that the term should not be used at all. Oliver (2012) points to the tremendous diversity among new religions and says that even though some "so-called cults" meet the criteria defined by Lifton, there is "enormous variation in the structure, doctrine and practice of new religious movements". He cites evidence from research studies showing that being part of a new religious movement is a positive experience for many.

It is difficult to determine how much anti-cult sentiment exists because these groups challenge existing or political authority rather than because they are believed to have negative effects on their followers. Parents, for example, may be upset that an adult child has rejected the family's religion. Governments may be concerned that a group's beliefs or activities undermine their authority or inspire terrorism. In some cases, the line between anti-cultism and totalitarian oppression may be vague or nonexistent.

4.7 Religious and spiritual abuse

Like so many other terms used in this book, the terms "religious abuse" and "spiritual abuse" are hard to define and lack a single meaning. Oakley & Kinmond (2013) suggest that part of the reason for this may be that what constitutes abuse may be defined differently in diverse cultural contexts. Writing from a Christian perspective in the United Kingdom, they define spiritual abuse as coercion and control of one person by another in a spiritual context, whether well-intentioned or not. Spiritual abuse occurs when religious authority is used to dominate, exploit, manipulate, or abuse an individual or group. The Institute for Muslim Mental Health (Long, 2017) describes several ways in which spiritual or religious communities can foster abuse:

• Members of the community feel pressure to conform to the rules of a religious or spiritual authority or to their faith community to the detriment of their own well-being.

- Backlash from a faith community occurs when someone reports or makes public an incident of abuse.
- Religious or spiritual leaders exerting control over followers, often for personal aims or financial gain.

Simonic *et al.* (2013) point out that while religious beliefs can be a positive influence on family life, they can also foster and justify abusive behaviors. In their review of the scant literature on religious abuse in the family, they describe two kinds of research. The first is research on partner abuse and the second is research on child abuse. As far as spousal abuse is concerned, they found that religious differences between spouses heighten the risk of spousal abuse. In particular, men with more conservative religious beliefs than their partners are more likely to be physically abusive toward them. With respect to religious child abuse, they identify the following:

- Medical neglect due to religious beliefs[3]
- Abuse committed by people with religious authority, and
- Abuse intended to purge children of evil

Abuse may be physical or emotional or both. Common forms of abuse mentioned by the authors are:

> spurning (rejecting or degrading behavior), terrorizing (threatening injury, death, or abandonment), isolating (refusing opportunities to interact), exploiting/corrupting (encouraging engagement in inappropriate behaviors), and denying emotional responsiveness (ignoring human needs for interaction and affection" (p. 341). The caregiver may not have the conscious intention of harming the child when manifesting these behaviors, in fact they may believe that they are helping the child, but Simonic and her coauthors point out that these behaviors may convey to the child that they are "worthless, flawed, unloved, unwanted, endangered, or only of value in meeting another's needs" (*ibid*).

The National FGM Centre is a UK non-profit organization dedicated to protecting children from female genital mutilation and other harmful practices. One of their foci is child abuse that is linked to faith or belief. They

---

[3] Some states in the U.S. have exemptions making parents exempt from responsibility for obtaining certain medical procedures for their children if their religion forbids it.

offer a list that includes several different religious folk beliefs that can put children at risk for abuse. Included in the list are the following beliefs:

- Spirit possession, demons or the devil acting through children or leading them astray (traditionally seen in some Christian beliefs).
- The evil eye or evil spirits (for example, djinns in Islamic folk religion and dakinis in Hindu or Buddhist contexts).
- Ritual murders where the killing of children is believed to bring supernatural benefits or the use of their body parts is believed to produce potent magical remedies (for example, "muti" murders in South Africa).
- The use of belief in magic or witchcraft to create fear in children to make them more compliant when they are being trafficked for domestic slavery or sexual exploitation.

The United Nations Children's Fund (UNICEF) has called on religious communities to take a leadership role in ending violence against children, issuing the following statement in 2010:

> We must acknowledge that our religious communities have not fully upheld their obligations to protect our children from violence. Through omission, denial and silence, we have at times tolerated, perpetuated and ignored the reality of violence against children in homes, families, institutions and communities, and not actively confronted the suffering that this violence causes. Even as we have not fully lived up to our responsibilities in this regard, we believe that religious communities must be part of the solution to eradicating violence against children, and we commit ourselves to take leadership in our religious communities and the broader society.

Shupe (2007) has observed that religious groups and institutions, because they are hierarchical systems characterized by unequal power and command the trust of their members, are especially prone to the abuse of their spiritual authority. Global public outrage over the failure of religious organizations to respond to reports of sexual abuse by clergy has received much attention in recent decades and placed pressure on religious leaders to respond more vigorously. This is not just a Western phenomenon. Women in Muslim countries have created their own #MosqueMeToo movement and there are Buddhist #MeToo movements in China and other Asian countries. In June of 2021, Pope Francis revised the Catholic Church's definition of sexual abuse to "explicitly acknowledge that adults, and not only children, can be victimized by priests and powerful laypeople who abuse their offices" and to criminalize their behavior (Horowitz, 2021). Despite the publicity, sexual abuse remains a problem across religions and spiritual orientations. Fortune, a Christian minister, and Enger, a rabbi, have discussed ways in which the Abrahamic religions can be used to justify violence against women (2005). Because they were written from the patriarchal perspective that characterized agrarian societies, both the Hebrew and Christian scriptures contain many passages confirming male dominance over women and telling stories about violence against women. Muslim sacred texts also have been interpreted by some as supportive of male dominance. The Institute for Muslim Mental Health (Long, 2017) urges mental health professionals to be aware of the following three behavioral indicators of abuse by spiritual authority figures:

1. The client shows signs of being intimidated by or afraid of their religious leader.
2. The person has withdrawn suddenly from their religious beliefs or community.
3. The client rationalizes the unacceptable behavior of the authority figure.

This is true although the sacred writings of all three religions prescribe kindness and compassion. Hindu texts also support male dominance and female submission and are used by some to condone domestic violence.

Religious abuse is often a component of colonization as part of an attempt to destroy indigenous cultures and replace them with the culture of the occupying power. Colonial empires have figured in human history since at least the 4th century BCE (Adams, 1984). The modern colonial era, however, is considered to have begun with the establishment of Spanish colonies in the Americas in the late 15th century.

4.8 Religious prejudice and persecution

Religious prejudice can be defined as a negative attitude toward those who hold different religious beliefs, are members of a group that holds particular religious beliefs, or who hold no religious beliefs at all. Burch-Brown & Baker (2016) have reviewed the literature on the relationship between religiosity and prejudice and found that the two are positively correlated, although the strength of the relationship seems to be decreasing over time. Religious prejudice often is a sign of deeper economic, ethnic, or political conflict and can be used to justify discrimination and persecution directed toward particular groups. Religious prejudice has often been used by colonial powers to stamp out indigenous religions and by totalitarian governments to eliminate any religion at all. The Pew Research Center (2020b) has found that harassment of religious groups continues to be reported in more than 90% of countries. As might be expected, religious restrictions are most common in authoritarian countries. Religious tolerance is a relatively modern notion and religious freedom is still not a basic right in many countries, though religious freedom is protected by international law, notably by actions of the United Nations. Bothwell (2019) points out that:

> The United Nations system has generated an array of international conventions, covenants, and resolutions which today articulate the rights of adherents to all sects and no sect. Religious freedom — sometimes used as shorthand for freedom of religion, belief, and conscience, is spelled out in the International Covenant on Civil and Political Rights, the 1981 Declaration on the Elimination of All Forms of Intolerance and of Discrimination Based on Religion or Belief, and other progeny of the U.N. Charter (p. 1).

Most recently, the United Nations Human Rights Council has adopted a resolution (2011) requiring member nations to combat "intolerance, negative stereotyping and stigmatization of, and discrimination of, incitement to violence and violence against, persons based on religion or belief." Research suggests that religious organizations and their clergy play an important role in promoting religious tolerance (Kalin & Siddiqui, 2014).

The First Amendment to the U.S. Constitution protects religious freedom and Title VII of the U.S. Civil Rights Act of 1964 prohibits employers from discriminating against individuals based on their religious beliefs (or lack thereof) in hiring, firing, or any other terms and conditions of employment. Also, it requires employers to make reasonable accommodations for the beliefs and practices of employees, including adjustments that would permit employees to practice their religion or to follow the dress and grooming rules of their religion. In spite of this legislation, the American Civil Liberties Union (n.d.) reports that it is seeing, with increasing frequency, individuals and institutions in the U.S. claiming the right to discriminate based on religious objections. Some of the forms that this discrimination can take include:

- Religiously affiliated schools firing unmarried women who became pregnant.
- Business owners refusing to provide insurance coverage for contraception for their employees.
- Graduate students, training to be social workers, refusing to counsel people who are LGBT.
- Pharmacies turning away women seeking to fill birth control prescriptions.
- Bridal salons, photo studios, and reception halls closing their doors to same-sex couples planning weddings.

Most countries have some form of legislation and/or oversight committee to prevent discrimination based on religion but the Pew Research Foundation reports that 28% of countries in 2018 placed high or very high restrictions on religion (Pew Research Center, 2020b). The same study revealed that 42% of countries have a state religion or preferred religion (a religion afforded preferential treatment by the government).

A 2016 Pew Research Center survey of 198 countries (Kushi, 2018) found that more than a quarter (28%) of the countries had "high" or "very high" levels of government restriction on religion. The survey asked about 20 indicators of government restrictions, including limits on proselytizing or public preaching and detentions or assaults of religious group members. A similar percentage of countries (27%) were rated as "high" or "very high" on measures of social hostilities involving religion, including tensions between religious groups and religion-related terrorism. Another Pew Research Center report (Lipka & Majumdar, 2019) showed that while interreligious tension and violence declined globally between 2001 and 2017, government restrictions on religion increased during these years in the four categories studied. Types of restriction include:

- Favoritism of religious groups
- General laws and policies restricting religious freedom
- Harassment of religious groups
- Limits on religious activity

Indonesia is a Muslim country that permits to a degree freedom to certain religions but has strong limits on that freedom. It recognizes only six religions: Islam, Protestantism, Catholicism, Hinduism, Buddhism, and Confucianism. Each of these religions is governed by an appointed national council that defines the permissible beliefs and practices for that religion. Individuals can be prosecuted for deviation from acceptable beliefs and practices and can serve up to five years in prison if convicted.

We tend to think that liberal Western democracies such as Norway also allow full religious freedom, but this is not necessarily the case, especially for religious minorities. Fox (2020) points out that Norway engages in substantial restrictions on religious minorities. Laws governing the slaughter of animals, for example, ban the ritual slaughter of meat as dictated by Judaism and Islam. It is often difficult to obtain building permits for mosques and burial requirements are such that not all Muslim burial customs are permitted. Head coverings cannot cover the face, even partially, in Norwegian public schools and universities. Such restrictions are common in many Western democracies. Religious restrictions are much more draconian in countries with religious or explicitly anti-religious governments. The Sunni Muslim government of Saudi Arabia, for example, does not permit public worship by any religion other than Islam and the religious curriculum in schools disparages Sufi and Shia Muslim religious practices and considers Jews and Christians "unbelievers" with whom Muslims should not associate (Human Rights Watch, 2017). In the U.S., 75% of Muslims say there is a lot of discrimination against Muslims and 82% say that they have experienced specific instances of discrimination such as being treated with suspicion, singled out by airport security, or called offensive names.

The Pew Research Center (2020b) reports that in 2018, government restrictions on religion reached their highest level globally in more than a decade. This report found that authoritarian governments were more likely to restrict religion and found that harassment of religious groups was reported in over 90% of countries. Harassment was defined as anything from verbal abuse to physical violence and killings motivated at least in part by the target's religious identity. Christians, Muslims, and Jews were the most likely to be harassed. The authors distinguished between government harassment (government laws, policies, and actions that restrict religious beliefs and practices) and social harassment (acts of religious hostility by private individuals, organizations, or groups in society). Buddhist, Christians, Hindus, Muslims, and religiously unaffiliated people were most likely to be harassed by governments. Jews, on the other hand, experienced more social harassment.

Even when national governments condone or advocate religious intolerance, there are variations within countries. Sumaktoyo (2018), for example, has shown wide differences among Indonesian provinces in Muslims' intolerance of Christians. Karpov & Lisovskaya (2007) have also found regional differences in the extent to which Russian Orthodox Christians are intolerant of Muslims. Another study carried out in Indonesia has shown that, at an individual level, income and education are both positively correlated with tolerance while religiosity and living in an area with high levels of poverty are negatively correlated with tolerance (Yusuf *et al.*, 2020). Religious persecution is typically attributed to differences between a dominant religious group and a minority religious group, but it often has less to do with religion and much more to do with territory and political processes. A British ecumenical Christian group, the Joint Public Issues Team (n.d.), has identified three causes of religious persecution:

- State regulation of religious activities
- Nationalism: perceived threat of minority groups to dominant group
- Fundamentalism: a regime or movement that stresses literal adherence to a set of basic principles

It is important to bear in mind that most fundamentalism is benign and is not associated with religious extremism or violence of any kind. Pratt (2010) has distinguished among three types, or degrees, of **fundamentalism** ranging from the completely benign to the extremely dangerous. The first he calls "passive fundamentalism". It is characterized by what he calls "perspectival absolutism" and "immediate inerrancy". The fundamentalist perspective is absolute — no other perspectives are entertained — and the relevant texts or scriptures are without error. He calls the second type "assertive fundamentalism".

Assertive fundamentalism has all of the characteristics of passive fundamentalism along with four more. First, the only genuine knowledge is perceived as consisting of "facts" contained in the sacred texts or scriptures, all else (including conflicting scientific findings) being false. Second, the identity of the individual is inextricably connected to the identity of the fundamentalist community and the stronger or more hardline or assertive the community, the tighter the connection. Third, assertive fundamentalism excludes religious liberalism of any sort and, fourth, it is characterized by what he calls a "condemnatory stance" or "strident assertions of a condemnatory or judgmental sort".

"Impositional fundamentalism" is the most extreme sort of fundamentalism and involves the contemplation, advocacy, or actual carrying out of violence. The non-believer or "religious other" is often perceived as evil or satanic, justifying organized terrorism. A study of over 23,000 adults in Egypt, Iraq, Jordan, Lebanon, Pakistan, Saudi Arabia, Tunisia, and Turkey (Moaddel & Karabenick, 2018) shows that fundamentalism is stronger in countries where religious liberty is lower, religion less fractionalized, state structure less fragmented, regulation of religion greater, and the national context less globalized. Among individuals within countries, fundamentalism is linked to religiosity, confidence in religious institutions, belief in religious modernity, belief in conspiracies, xenophobia, fatalism, weaker liberal values, trust in family and friends, reliance on less diverse information sources, lower socioeconomic status, and membership in an ethnic majority or dominant religion/sect.

Gomes (2013) has found that religious intolerance in a country is positively related to the degree of civil conflict (organized armed conflict between groups in the same country). This was true even when he controlled for ethnic differences between religious groups. He also found that civil conflict was greater when there was more government regulation of religion. He found that the Abrahamic religions (Judaism, Christianity, and Islam) and Indian religions (most notably, Hinduism and Sikhism) were associated with a high degree of civil conflict. Schleutker (2020) has written about how authoritarian regimes use religion to reinforce and retain their power through co-opting strategically important groups and individuals in a society so that they have a vested interest in the survival of the regime. Negative restrictions on religion also strengthen the regime by enabling them to disempower and repress opposition by certain groups. The right to religious freedom can also help protect minority ethnic groups and other groups that might otherwise be persecuted for religious or political reasons. The Cleveland Council on World Affairs (2014) has pointed out that religious tolerance benefits individual countries as well as the international community, noting that countries that practice religious tolerance have higher than average economic growth, probably due to investor and tourist confidence both within and outside the country.

4.9 Violent religious extremism

Wibisono *et al.* (2019) have sought to bring clarity to the term "religious extremism", arguing that it is a multidimensional concept that is often oversimplified. They identify four dimensions relevant to religious extremism. Each dimension has two poles: a moderate pole and an extremist pole and many gradations in between. They apply this model to Muslim religious groups in Indonesia and demonstrate that there is great variation among these groups in where they fall on each of the four dimensions. The four dimensions are:

1. Theological
   - Moderate: Belief in the graciousness of God and appreciation of differences in beliefs
   - Extreme: Authoritarian image of God, hostility toward different beliefs
2. Ritual
   - Moderate: Rituals are traditions, variations are tolerated
   - Extreme: Rituals are given by God, purity must be maintained
3. Social
   - Moderate: Open to interreligious collaboration and internal change to solve problems
   - Extreme: Hostile view of other faiths, out-group blamed for in-group's problems
4. Political
   - Moderate: Desire to integrate religious values within the current political system
   - Extreme: Hope for an Islam state or empire governed by Sharia law[4]

---

[4] Sharia law: Islamic law derived from religious writings.

This is an especially useful deconstruction of the concept of religious extremism and the dimensions can be applied to other religious groups, though the definitions of "moderate" and "extreme" political extremism would have to be redefined to match the goals of each group. One limit of this model is that it does not include the dimension of violence, which is a key component of many extremist positions (Table 4.8). The World

Table 4.8.   Some examples of violent religious extremist organizations.

Groups	Description
The Army of God	A U.S. Christian anti-abortion terrorist organization that promotes killing abortion providers and attacking abortion clinics.
Eastern Lightning	A violently proselytizing Christian doomsday* cult that originated in China.
The Lord's Resistance Army	A Christian group founded in Uganda, which calls for a fundamentalist Christian government in that country with laws that are the Christian equivalent of Sharia law. It has committed thousands of killings and kidnappings and has spread to South Sudan, the Central African Republic, and the Democratic Republic of Congo.
The National Liberation Front of Tripura	A paramilitary, anti-Hindu, Christian organization based in Tripura, India. It began and was, at least initially, supported by a Baptist church. It is known for attacks on Hindus who refuse to convert to their extreme form of Protestant fundamentalism.
Al Qaeda	A loosely organized, multinational collection of militant fundamentalist Sunni Islamist groups advocating the creation of an Islamic state in Iraq and Syria and the elimination of all foreigners from Muslim countries. It began with the anti-Soviet jihad** in Afghanistan in the 1980s and subsequently joined with other militant extremist Muslim groups. It has been responsible for terrorist attacks and bombings, including the September 11th attacks on the World Trade Center in New York in 2001. It was led by Osama bin Laden until 2011, when he was killed by U.S. military forces in Pakistan.
Islamic State of Iraq and Syria (ISIS)	ISIS is also a fundamentalist Sunni Islamist jihadist organization that began in Iraq. It has the goal of establishing a Sunni Islamic State in Iraq and the Levant (an area including parts of Lebanon and Jordan). It has been responsible for multiple attacks and bombings including the 2015 Charlie Hebdo magazine massacre carried out in reaction to a cartoon caricaturing the prophet Mohammed.

Table 4.8.   (*Continued*)

Groups	Description
Taliban	The Taliban are an Afghan, primarily Sunni, Islamic group who returned to power in Afghanistan in 2021. During their previous rule between 1996 and 2001 they were known for their terrorism, oppression, and violent enforcement of Sharia law.
Rashtriya Swayamsevak Sangh (RSS)	RSS is an Indian, pro-Hindu, paramilitary organization that has been involved in riots and anti-Muslim violence but that also advocates social reform and has been involved in social welfare work, including providing masks and food during the 2020 coronavirus lockdown in India.

*Prophesying the end of the world, apocalyptic.
**A jihad is a holy war on behalf of Islam that is seen as a religious obligation.

Economic Forum (Muggah & Velshi, 2019) has expressed alarm at the rise in violent religious tensions in the past decade, ranging from "Islamic extremists waging global jihad and power struggles between Sunni and Shia Muslims in the Middle East to the persecution of Rohingya in Myanmar and outbreaks of violence between Christians and Muslims across Africa" (p. 1). They argue that interfaith cooperation is required to reduce religious violence, citing a long history of peaceful solutions that emerged from collaboration among faith-based groups and their leaders. Kakar (2020) has pointed to the destructive power of a communal "religious identity" that is organized around religious affiliation and is characterized by exclusivity, intolerance, and a potential for violence against other "enemy" groups. He advocates for a massive educational effort for children to counteract family and community influences that produce religious violence.

This chapter has only skimmed the surface of its subject: the many forms of religious expression, both positive and negative. Its purpose was to orient the reader to the range of religious affiliations that exist. In clinical practice, it is necessary in each case to acquire more in-depth knowledge about each client's religious beliefs and practices from that client and, in many cases, it is necessary to do further research. It can be helpful to visit websites related to the client's religion or the religious organization to which they belong, or to read articles or books about the religion. Dudley (2016) also suggests learning about interfaith groups in your area that may be sponsoring events where you can learn more about various religions. An excellent reference book that discusses the implications for psychotherapy of a number of religious denominations and sects is *Handbook of Psychotherapy and Religious Diversity* by Richards & Bergin (2014).

Discussion questions

1. Do you belong to any faith groups or organizations?

2. How would you describe yourself in terms of your religiosity?

3. If you belong to a religion, are there groups or categories of people against which it is prejudiced?

4. Do you think it is necessary to agree with a client's religious point of view to support it?

5. Are there any religious biases or stereotypes you hold?

Exercises

1. Watch this video about the five major religions and describe your reaction in one paragraph: https://www.youtube.com/watch?v=m6d Cxo7t_aE

2. Take this "religious typology test": https://www.pewforum.org/quiz/religious-typology/. Do you feel that the type you were characterized by in the test is accurate? Why or why not? What kinds of biases, if any, do you see in this test?

3. Watch this video, "Misunderstandings about Religion". Describe your reaction in one paragraph: https://www.openculture.com/2018/03/harvard-launches-a-free-online-course-to-promote-religious-tolerance-understanding.html

Resource

The Yale Divinity School Library website offers a guide to free resources on religion at: https://guides.library.yale.edu/c.php?g=295851&p=1972637

Chapter 5

Spirituality and Human Development

The field of human development is concerned with how individuals change and grow and with the genetic, biological, psychological, social, and cultural patterns and structures that influence their development. The discipline grew out of long-term studies of children's growth and behavior that began in the 1930s. As behavioral scientists began to acknowledge that we continue to develop and learn throughout life, the field of human development expanded beyond child development into the adult years and old age. Even the process of death has been viewed from a developmental perspective (Kübler-Ross, 2011). Most theories of human development stress the impact of early experience on later development and adult personality. They also assume that the ability to cope positively with any particular developmental issue depends in part on the extent to which an individual has coped positively with prior developmental issues.

Developmental theories are optimistic. They see growth and development as the natural tendency of the organism as it interacts with its environment. Even when environmental circumstances are less than ideal, individuals do their best to learn and grow, often showing considerable resilience. The degree to which an individual manifests resilience reflects both genetic and environmental factors as well as their learned ability to cope. The often-used term, "**developmental stage**", indicates that individuals at similar points in the life cycle often have similar concerns, perceptions, feelings, or techniques for coping, even if their personalities are quite different from one another. At each stage, they face certain common developmental or "socio-emotional" tasks (Erikson, 1980). The resolution of the **developmental task**, or crisis, at any one stage in development provides a foundation for the successful resolution of later ones. Someone who is not able to resolve the developmental crisis that characterizes one stage may be at a disadvantage when confronting the challenges of a later stage. Most well-known theories of human development reflect an Anglo-European worldview, but other cultural contexts and perspectives will also be discussed in this section.

The ongoing popularity of Erikson's conceptualization of developmental stages bears witness to its usefulness, despite its limitations. Stage theories are helpful in therapy because they draw a therapist's attention to past, present, and future age-related challenges and concerns but are often misused in practice. Focusing uncritically on age-related stages can cause the therapist to miss significant differences among clients of similar ages. Stage theories also imply an invariant linear process in development while this is not necessarily the case. There are individual and cultural differences in the nature and order of stages of psychosocial development. Development is not necessarily unidirectional. Individuals may revisit earlier stages or manifest the characteristics of more than one stage at the same time. No developmental task is ever permanently resolved — similar issues may crop up across the life cycle. Also, trauma at any age, but particularly in childhood, may disrupt development.

While most of the major theories of human development have originated in England, Europe, and North America, theorists and researchers from other parts of the world also have made important contributions. In addition, many of the world's religions are implicitly based on certain assumptions concerning life stages. For example, ancient Indian Vedic texts present a model of stages in development that is very similar to Erikson's (Rangaswami, 1992; Olson, 2002). Chakkarath (2013) has argued that it is important to include Indian thought in discussions about human development and, in general, to think about human development in a cross-cultural framework. He is a part of what has been called the "indigenous psychology movement", which advocates the scientific study of human emotions and behavior in the culture in which they naturally occur rather than transporting theory and research from one region to another (Kim & Berry, 1993). Life-stage transitions are often acknowledged and celebrated by societies, communities, or families, in what are called "**rites of passage**" (van Gennep, 1960). For example, initiation rites are common, especially for males, in pre-literate societies and many religions, ancient and modern, to mark the transition from adolescence to adulthood.

Feiler (2021) has written a stinging critique of stage theories. He argues that life transitions are not linear or predictable as stage theorists would have us believe. Instead, they are caused by disrupting events, or "lifequakes". Feiler's book, *Life is in the Transitions*, is worth reading because it is provocative and counters too-literal applications of stage theories. On the other hand, he focuses on major "lifequakes" and ignores the importance of neurobiological development and the common life transitions that contribute to shared resources and challenges in each age range. Also, ironically, in spite of his objections to stage theories, he cannot help offering a linear stage theory of transition. The stages are: the long goodbye, the messy middle, and the new beginning. Judith Viorst in her book, *Necessary Losses* (1998), points out that while each stage of development offers new possibilities, development also results in losses. Birth, itself, creates loss because it involves the infant's loss of "oneness" with the mother.

5.1 Infancy

The birth of a child is an important event in family and community life and many religious and spiritual traditions have ceremonies to mark this occasion. Some examples are baptism in the Christian faith, naming in Judaism, and Shahadah in Islam. In China, a naming ceremony was traditionally held for male babies at one month, but this tradition has since expanded to include female babies as well. Secular ceremonies also are held by many families to celebrate a child's birth.

The concept of **attachment** is central to describing development in infancy and attachment is considered by many to be the foundation for spirituality. Attachment theory (Cassidy, 1999; Mooney, 2009) was originally formulated by John Bowlby (1983), and further developed by Mary Ainsworth (1964). Ainsworth's original studies were carried out in Uganda and later in the U.S. Its central premise is that normal social and emotional development depends on the development of a secure and unbroken attachment to at least one **parenting figure**[1] in infancy and childhood. This attachment provides the child with a working model for other relationships,

---

[1]This term is used to apply to the child's primary caregiver(s), even if they are not the parents.

including a relationship with the spiritual or non-material realm. Continuity in the caregiver relationship and responsiveness on the part of the caregiver to the child's needs are essential for secure attachment. Young children with secure attachments show distress when their primary caregiver leaves them with a stranger, show pleasure and affection when the caregiver returns, and turn to the primary caregiver for comfort when distressed. Secure attachment in infancy predisposes an individual to go on to seek out and form positive relationships with others and can support their spiritual development. Griffith (2012) uses attachment theory to explain variation in how believers relate to God. A person who has a **secure attachment** style and believes in God is comforted by this belief when they are anxious because they feel that God is present and will respond if needed. A person with an **insecure/anxious attachment** style feels that God, though strong and capable, may not be reliably available, perhaps because they do not feel worthy of God's attention. Such a believer may focus on placating God and praying for help. A person who expects little from God and cultivates self-reliance may have an **avoidant attachment** style. Griffith argues that a secure attachment to a personal God acts as a potent buffer against demoralization. A predisposition to secure attachment can be reassuring without a belief in a deity, however, since, as we shall see, it leads to what Erikson calls "basic trust".

Erik Erikson, a psychoanalytically trained psychiatrist (1980), laid the groundwork for the approach known as **ego psychology** and popularized one of the most influential stage theories of human development. He initially described eight stages in development and later, with his wife Joan Erikson, added a ninth (Erikson & Erikson, 1998). Erikson's stages build on Sigmund Freud's **psychosexual** theory of development, which emphasized sexual, or libidinal, maturation and its effects on the development of the psyche. Freud conceptualized a tripartite organization of the psyche consisting of the id (sexual and other urges), the superego (the conscience), and the ego (actor in the world and mediator between id and ego). The id is characterized by what Freud called "primary process thinking", a kind of preverbal, illogical thinking that occurs in dreams and focuses on immediate wish-fulfillment. He disparaged mystical or transcendental experience, which he called "oceanic feeling", as infantile. Erikson was most concerned with the ego and how it is shaped by the twin influences of the id and its social environment, but unlike Freud, he had a positive perspective on spirituality. Like Freud, however, he believed that unconscious psychological processes shape much of our thought and behavior. Though developmental theorists and researchers still draw on his work, Erikson wrote in the 1950s and 1960s from the standpoint of a European-American. As a result, many of his conceptualizations are dated and limited by his perspective.

The first, and most essential, Eriksonian stage is known as **Basic Trust vs. Mistrust**. The infant begins life without a sense of "self and other" and gradually learns this distinction through interaction with its physical and social environment. Along with the recognition of oneself as a separate being, this stage involves attachment to a parenting figure. If the infant experiences nurturing and reliable caregiving, they will develop what Erikson calls "a basic sense of trust in life and the universe". As for other stages, this is not an either/or dichotomy but rather an attitudinal continuum between trust and mistrust that may vary over time as new developmental challenges emerge. Only the roughest of age ranges can be given for any stage, since different sources give different ages and individuals mature at widely different rates. The period during which a sense of basic trust is typically achieved (or not) is during the first 18 months to 2 years of life. Many developmental psychologists see infancy as a **critical period** for the development of trust, meaning that if attachment and trust are not accomplished in this phase, their eventual attainment may be seriously jeopardized. Porges (2019) sees the development of attachment and trust during this period as the foundation for spiritual development. In 1989, after the Romanian dictator Nicolae Ceaușescu was executed, it was quickly learned that vast numbers of children were being raised in orphan asylums where they experienced severe neglect and a lack of opportunity to form attachments to their caregivers. Nelson *et al.* (2013) compared children who were moved to foster homes to those who remained in orphanages and found that, while their development lagged behind that of children who had never been institutionalized, those who had been placed in foster homes did better than those who remained in institutions. Those who had been placed into foster care before the age of two showed the most improvement.

The DSM-5 defines a trauma-related condition of early childhood that results from maltreatment and neglect. It is called **Reactive Attachment Disorder** and is characterized by a lack of positive attachment behaviors, rapid mood changes, inconsolability, behavior problems, delayed motor development, and impaired cognitive functioning (Ellis, Yilanli, & Saabadi, 2021). Children who experience foster care, adoption, or institutional care are particularly vulnerable to this condition because the separations involved can disrupt or prevent the primary attachment experience that is so important in development. There is no strong empirical evidence indicating the effectiveness of any particular method for treating Reactive Attachment Disorder and some, such as holding therapy, have been rejected by mental health professional organizations in the U.S. and other countries (Mercer, 2014). Holding therapy consists of the forcible holding of a child by a parent or therapist until the child relaxes and stops resisting.

Cultures differ in terms of the ways and extent to which they promote an attitude of trust in infants. Gregg (2005) describes the "pediatric" model of infant care used in most of sub-Saharan Africa, South Asia, and many pre-industrial societies. This model is suitable for environments in which the survival of the infant is at risk and involves nearly continuous physical contact, immediate soothing of distress, and long-term, on-demand breastfeeding. It may involve the sharing of a "family bed". This maximizes the infant's chances of survival while minimizing the likelihood of another pregnancy. Gregg argues that it is also especially conducive to the formation of a sense of basic trust. Pediatric infant care contrasts with the "pedagogic" model, more common in industrial and post-industrial societies. In these societies, the survival of the infant tends to be taken for granted and face-to-face social interaction and education are prioritized with the aim of promoting the infant's social and intellectual development. Gregg (*ibid*) also points to differences between the pediatric and the pedagogic models with respect to how weaning is carried out. In industrial and post-industrial societies weaning is gradual and households typically consist of only the nuclear family. In pre-industrial societies, weaning is more abrupt and accompanied by a decrease in maternal attention, often because of the birth of another child and the expectation that the young child will be cared for by siblings and other members of the extended family. Gregg argues that the pediatric model is especially supportive of autonomy because the infant must learn independence and techniques for reaching out to an array of relatives for nurturing. It could also be argued, however, that abrupt weaning with a sudden decrease in maternal attention could detract from the trust that had been established earlier.

Jean Piaget, a Swiss psychologist, formulated a stage theory of cognitive development (1977) that spread widely in the 1960s. It complements Erikson's work by giving a fuller picture of cognitive development during infancy, childhood, and adolescence and argues that learning is not just a matter of absorbing more information but rather a process in which the child's thinking undergoes specific qualitative changes. Lawrence Kohlberg, an American psychologist, extended Piaget's work on the moral judgments of children to develop a comprehensive stage theory of moral development (1984). Cross-cultural research has not always supported his research findings, however. For example, Baek (2002) found that the responses of Korean children to Kohlberg's moral judgment tasks did not always fit into the response categories given in Kohlberg's coding manual, suggesting that there were some traditional Chinese concepts that Kohlberg was not aware of. Piaget calls cognitive development in infancy the **Sensorimotor** stage. At this point, infants are already miniature scientists, noticing sounds, physical sensations, and the effects of their movements and actions. They learn that they are a separate entity from objects and other people in their environment and that their behavior has consequences. They also develop a concept of object permanence, or the knowledge that people or objects exist even when they cannot see them. Peekaboo is a game that specially delights infants who are in the process of developing a sense of object permanence. When the infant knows that their parent or caregiver still exists even when they are away, it is easier to adjust to their periodic absence. Toward the end of the first two years, children begin to use symbols, including language and images, and are aware of gender. Most show a preference for toys considered appropriate for the gender they were assigned at birth but some already show a strong preference for toys associated with the "opposite" gender (quotation marks added because gender is not necessarily a dichotomous variable; there are many ways in which it can be defined).

Kohlberg does not speculate about the moral development of preverbal infants, but Van de Voort & Hamlin (2016) have suggested, based on a review of observational studies of infants, that even infants are able to distinguish between actions that are helpful and those that are harmful or hindering. The research shows that infants show a preference and pay more attention to individuals who they see as helpful. What makes this moral discernment, as opposed to just self-interest, is that, at 8 months, the infants studied preferred individuals who intended to help, regardless of whether they succeeded or not, over individuals who intended to harm or hinder. The authors call this **Intuitive Morality**.

Fowler (1995), a Methodist minister and professor of Theology and Human Development, built on Erikson's, Piaget's, and Kohlberg's work to create a stage theory of spiritual development. Fowler's stages have to do with what, from his Christian perspective, he calls "faith development". For him, faith is a belief in God or a higher power. It is, however, still consistent with his paradigm to interpret faith as an expanded basic trust that includes a sense that the universe is safe, and that life and death make sense and have meaning. Fowler refers to an infant's spiritual orientation as **Undifferentiated Faith**, which is basically the same thing as Erikson's basic trust.

In summary, developments that typically occur in infancy and that provide a foundation for spirituality are: attachment, trust, a sense of self and other, and an awareness of cause and effect.

5.2 Early childhood

For Erikson, there are two developmental stages in early childhood. The first is **Autonomy vs. Shame and Doubt,** which occurs roughly between one to three years. The term autonomy denotes a "sense of self-control without a loss of self-esteem" (Erikson, 1980, p. 70). The child is more mobile and independent, encountering limit-setting from parenting figures and others and frequently hearing the word "no" during attempts to explore and manipulate a newly accessible world. Toilet training, which usually begins during this period, can result in feelings of shame and self-doubt, depending on the empathy and severity with which it is imposed and the child's ability to control elimination as expected. While this stage challenges a child's sense of self-worth, a child who is securely attached and respectfully treated will eventually learn to use the toilet and will develop a feeling of autonomy based on what Bandura has called a sense of "**self-efficacy**". Bandura (1997) defines self-efficacy as a belief "in one's capabilities to organize and execute the course of action required to produce given attainments" (p. 3).

Erikson's second childhood stage is **Initiative vs. Guilt** and occurs roughly between the ages of three and six. During this stage, children are becoming much more independent and, at the same time, admire and are eager to be like their parents. While they cannot yet take on adult roles or privileges, they do begin to internalize many of their parents' attitudes, including a sense of right and wrong, or a conscience. The task in this stage is to internalize and conform to cultural standards for behavior while maintaining a proactive attitude toward the future and without being hamstrung by excessive guilt. While parents with a more egalitarian orientation may avoid inducing undue feelings of guilt in their children, they may be less effective at helping their children form a strong conscience. More authoritarian parenting styles, however, may be more effective in producing strong consciences in children but also may install a more limiting sense of guilt. Experts typically recommend an authoritative parenting style. This type of parenting is characterized by clear limits, warmth, and measured consequences for misbehavior that are explained to the child by the parent (Baumrind, 2013).

Piaget points to the importance of the acquisition of language and symbolic thought in late infancy and early childhood because these capabilities will later permit abstract thought. However, children's thought in early childhood is still very primitive and concrete. He calls this period "preoperational", meaning that young children are not able to reason logically. This can result in what has been called "**magical thinking**", or the belief that two unrelated events are causally connected. For example, a child may believe that putting salt on food cools the food or that some thought of theirs has brought harm to a parent. Early childhood thinking is egocentric — though children recognize that they are separate beings from others, they are not yet able to imagine or take into account a perspective different from their own. For example, they may not recognize how a model of a mountain would look from the other side of a table (one of the tasks Piaget used in studying cognitive development). They also may not recognize that some changes, for example death, are permanent, and may not assume, as most older individuals do, that gender identity is expected to be stable throughout life. Of course, thanks to activism by LGBT activists and others, many adolescents and adults now recognize that gender identity does not, in fact, necessarily remain stable over time.

For Kohlberg, moral development begins in early childhood. He calls the first level of moral development **Preconventional Morality**. This level has two stages. In the first, **Obedience and Punishment**, the child's thinking is, in Piaget's terms, egocentric. Children think about behavior in terms of its consequences for themselves. A behavior is good if it does not result in reprimand or punishment. A behavior is bad if it does. They believe that standards for right and wrong are absolute and are decided by an outside authority — their parents, a teacher, or perhaps even God. In the next stage, **Individualism and Exchange**, children begin to recognize that there is not just one single code of right and wrong created by an absolute authority but that different individuals (or households) have different viewpoints. They become aware they can often meet their own needs by engaging in reciprocal exchanges such as sharing or taking turns. Fowler applies these same concepts to spiritual development, labeling his early childhood stage **Intuitive-Projective**. In this egocentric stage, children are not capable of imagining perspectives other than their own and simply assume that their perspective is the only one. Their reasoning is imaginative rather than logical and their beliefs and values consist of those internalized through contact with parental adults. Children's growing imaginations and ability to think symbolically result in more anxieties and a fear of death, particularly parental death. He cites Bettelheim's work describing how stories such as fairy tales can help children externalize their fears and imagine conquering them.

Though children in early childhood are still limited by egocentric thinking and an inability to imagine perspectives other than their own, they are learning that they can meet their own needs through engaging in reciprocal activities. Developments that typically occur in early childhood and that provide a foundation for later spiritual development are language acquisition, causal (sometimes "magical") thinking, and a desire to avoid punishment.

5.3 Childhood

Erikson calls his childhood stage, which begins at around six years of age, **Industry vs. Inferiority**. This is a time when adults usually start introducing children to the basic skills they will need as adults in their society. It ends around the beginning of puberty, or about 12 or 13. While instruction in early pre-literate societies involves informal, person-to-person learning, literate societies are characterized by structured educational systems with increasingly specialized learning required at each ascending grade level. Indigenous children today may participate both in tribal learning and in required institutionalized learning. Colonial systems have often used educational institutions to eliminate tribal cultures, including languages, and to compel indigenous children to adopt the dominant culture.[2] Children often "play at" adult roles during this period, and internalize many of the beliefs, values, and attitudes of significant adults in their lives. They envy adults their rights and privileges but must learn to accept the fact that they must wait until they are older to qualify for them themselves. Their task at this time is to learn to work hard to complete tasks, master skills, and become competent. The risk is that the child will develop a sense of inadequacy and inferiority. The risk is greater when the school context is not supportive, or the child is not able to succeed due to inherent limitations such as ADHD and/or learning disabilities, or due to family and environmental circumstances. Racial, ethnic, and other forms of discrimination and sexism or homophobia may shape the child's school experience, resulting in feelings of inferiority. Children whose gender identity or erotic orientations are not consistent with social expectations may experience distress in childhood and some express a desire to transition to a different gender identity.

Piaget calls childhood the stage of **Concrete Operations**. In this stage, children begin to think logically and in a more organized fashion about concrete events and to form general principles based on their observations. They also develop the ability to look at things from an alternative perspective and to imagine how other people think and feel. George Herbert Mead contrasts the preschool child's "playing at" roles to the school-aged child's participation in games, which are organized systems of roles and require an awareness, not only of one's own role, but also the roles of other participants. This extends to the child's social experience as the child becomes able to understand relationships among social roles and develops a sense of the "**generalized other**", the perspective taken on when someone tries to imagine what others expect of them (Mead, 1934). While they can reason well about concrete reality, children in this stage still have difficulty with abstract, probabilistic, and hypothetical concepts. Kohlberg calls the level of moral development that emerges during this period **Conventional Morality**. The first stage at this

---

[2]The discovery in 2021 of numerous unmarked child graves at former residential schools for indigenous Canadian children has stimulated widespread outrage at the abuse and neglect that characterized such schools.

level is **Good Boy, Nice Girl**. In this stage, the child is motivated to conform to social expectations (the generalized other) regarding right and wrong so that they will be rewarded and seen as a good person by others. The feminist Gilligan (1982) has criticized Kohlberg's portrayal of Conventional Morality, pointing out that his research was conducted on males only and his conclusions reflect a logical and individualistic male perspective that emphasizes justice and rights and that makes women seem deficient by contrast. Instead, she proposes a feminist perspective that focuses on moral decisions regarding the care of self and others. She, in turn, has been criticized (e.g., Senchuk, 1990), also from a feminist perspective, because her "feminine voice" regards women's role solely in terms of caregiving and because she ignores the fact that men also must make decisions about caring for self and others.

Fowler adds a deeper dimension to Kohlberg's Good Boy, Nice Girl stage by naming this stage **Mythic-Literal Faith**. In this stage, through hearing and reading myths and stories, children begin to internalize on many of the beliefs and values portrayed in the literature of their society or subculture. Bettelheim (1975), in his book about the meaning and value of fairy tales, explores this topic from a Freudian perspective, arguing that fairy tales help children understand and cope with such upsetting feelings as anger, fear, jealousy, resentment, anxiety about their death or the death of their parents. Children are now vulnerable to what has been called "**moral injury**" (Norman & Maguen, n.d.). Moral injury can occur when someone does something that is not in line with their beliefs (commission) or they fail to do something that is in line with their beliefs (omission). Witnessing violence in the home or elsewhere is something that can cause moral injury in children because they have internalized the belief that it is wrong to hurt people but still have enough magical thinking going on to imagine they could have helped, even when helping would have been dangerous or impossible. Trauma expert Bessel van der Kolk (2009) has argued for the addition of a diagnosis of "**Developmental trauma disorder**" to the DSM to be used for children and adolescents exposed to chronic interpersonal trauma.

Developments that typically occur in childhood and that provide a foundation for later spiritual development are the desire to please others by being good and, later, the internalization of conventional beliefs and values. They also become capable of logical thinking but only in a very concrete way — they cannot yet understand probabilistic or hypothetical thinking.

5.4 Adolescence

Brain maturation produces marked progress in the ability of adolescents to reason and think abstractly while, at the same time, hormonal changes and sexual maturation can interfere with behavior regulation. According to Erikson, the next stage, **Identity vs. Identity Confusion**, extends from around the age of 12 to 19 years old, but views about the duration of adolescence have changed since Erikson's time. A Columbia University psychiatrist (Stetka, 2017) has been quoted as saying "25 is the new 18" because young adults have come to marry and achieve financial independence later than in earlier years. Recent research has indicated that the brain is not fully mature until sometime in the mid-20s (Arain *et al.*, 2013).

Adolescence marks the transition from childhood to adulthood. It involves the formation of a stable sense of oneself and one's identity, both internally and as projected to others. Up to this point, the individual has acquired many skills and played many roles. Now, they must sort through their past, present, and possible future identifications to integrate them and to become confident about who they are and who they want to become. This period is formative for expectations about education and occupational aspirations. Erikson reminds us that the successful resolution of earlier developmental tasks makes identity formation easier. At the same time, the adolescent in this stage may revisit earlier developmental tasks and need to resolve them anew. The risk in this stage is that the adolescent may not be able to develop a stable sense of identity that will lead to the formation and achievement of realistic goals and will flounder in the attempt to achieve a responsible adult standpoint. Again, sexism, racism, ethnocentrism, and other such "-isms" affect the ease or difficulty with which an adolescent can develop a positive and stable sense of identity. Romantic or erotic attachments provide ways for adolescents to explore their sexual identities and gender orientations and adolescents who recognize that they are gay, lesbian, transgendered, or members of other stigmatized sexual or gender categories can face a challenge integrating this knowledge with their other identities. Furthermore, they often lack guidance and support from responsible adults in this regard. "Coming out", or revealing one's true gender identity or sexual orientation, can cause conflict with parents or others or result in neighborhood or school bullying. A term that is used by some to refer to the incomplete resolution of the developmental task of identity formation is **developmental arrest**. Developmental arrest is a concept that originated in Freudian theory with the notion of "fixation" in a particular developmental stage and means that an individual, whether because of inherent limitations, trauma, or inadequate environmental support, has not been able to resolve the challenge of a particular stage and is therefore compromised with respect to the resolution of future developmental issues and may, when stressed, regress to the stage at which the fixation occurred.

For Piaget, the final stage in cognitive development, **Formal Operations**, begins in adolescence. The adolescent becomes able to think abstractly, to use logic to understand and solve hypothetical problems, and reason deductively from a general principle to an actual situation. In Kohlberg's framework, the second stage of Conventional Morality, **Law and Order**, is typically completed during adolescence. It requires abstract reasoning and involves an awareness that rules and laws exist to protect the social order, not just because violating them is punished or results in social disapproval. At this stage, the individual recognizes that maintaining the social order benefits everyone. The orientation is still toward authority and fixed rules but with greater understanding of their rationale and purpose. Kohlberg's belief that many adults never develop past this stage was confirmed in a study by van den Enden *et al.* (2019). They analyzed data from a massive study of moral development using an instrument known as the "Defining Issues Test", which was designed to measure stages of moral development. The study was based on responses from 55,319 adolescent and adult native English speakers, mostly from the U.S. and Canada. The study found that 55% of respondents had an average score of 4 (Law and Order) or below. Only 42% of the respondents scored at the Post-Conventional level (5 or 6), and only 3% scored at the highest level (6). Fowler's adolescent stage, **Synthetic-Conventional Faith**, is similar to Kohlberg's Law and Order stage in that it is made possible by the emergence of abstract reasoning ability and involves discerning the beliefs and values of one's immediate community, which are taken for granted rather than questioned or closely examined. Like Kohlberg, Fowler believes that many adults do not develop past this stage.

Joseph Campbell (2020) describes the function of initiation rites, which occur in many indigenous societies and other communities to mark the transition from adolescence to adulthood, as a "**hero journey**" and sees them as an enactment of the "monomyth", which underlies the story of the mythic hero. In this myth, the hero is suddenly called to leave the ordinary world and enter an alternate reality for an adventure that is dangerous or frightening. The hero is initially resistant but agrees after meeting a mentoring figure. The hero then enters a different world, experiences some kind of ordeal, and returns to the ordinary world with a treasure that can be used to help others. The experience bestows the hero with wisdom and power. Examples of the monomyth are the Pinocchio fairy tale, the Persephone myth, the bible story of Jonah in the belly of the whale, and the story of Jason and the Golden Fleece. Carl Jung refers to such heroes as "archetypes". An archetype is a model that represents certain universal human attributes and is portrayed or perceived as a mythic being. Relating to archetypal images can reveal to us personality traits of which we were previously unaware. Initiation rites usually involve some kind of test or ordeal such as circumcision, tattooing or scarification, or the recitation of sacred text, after which the adolescent is acknowledged as an adult by the community. Many spiritual and religious traditions have coming-of-age ceremonies that recognize the transition from childhood to adult responsibilities in society, for example confirmation in Christianity, the Bar or Bat Mitzvah in Judaism, the sacred thread ceremony in Hinduism, and Amrit Sanchar in Shintoism. Many of the indigenous North American tribes still honor the long-standing tradition of vision quests in which adolescents isolate themselves for a supernatural experience in which they seek to interact with a guardian spirit, usually an animal, to obtain protection and discern their **call**. Bankson (1999) has developed a cycle of stages that can take place when a person seeks their spiritual calling. Her stages are:

- **Resist:** Lack of trust in the call or in one's ability to fulfill it
- **Reclaim:** Reclaiming parts of oneself that have been buried or left behind
- **Revelation:** An event or insight that gives us clues to a new path
- **Risk:** Encounter with the "Poison River", the crucial crossing point where one chooses whether or not to proceed in spite of one's fears
- **Relate:** Making connections to others who will make the journey with us
- **Release:** A kind of generativity in which we pass on what we have accomplished or learned or let go of it in order to rest and open oneself to a new call

In summary, ideal development during adolescence involves the development of the ability to reason abstractly and the formation of a stable and positive sense of identity. While adolescents are still fairly conventional in their ideas of right and wrong, they are beginning to think critically about the beliefs and values that have been transmitted to them and to make choices among these and their alternatives that are consistent with their forming identities.

5.5 Adulthood

Erikson refers to the first adult stage as **Intimacy vs. Self-absorption**. Cultures differ in their expectations concerning intimacy and marriage. In many rural towns and villages of the world, especially Asia and sub-Saharan Africa, most women marry before they are 18 years old (UNICEF, 2020). In 2021, the average age at marriage in the U.S. was 28 for women and 30 for men (U.S. Census, 2021). Expectations in most cultures have also been changing over time. According to the United Nations Population Division (2016), global data show that both men and women are marrying later worldwide and are more likely to cohabit without marriage. Nonetheless, Roseneil and her co-authors (2020), based on a study of four quite different European countries, have coined the term "**couple-norm**", to refer to a set of norms that underlie the definition of adulthood in most parts of the world today. The couple-norm is a set of legal, social, and cultural norms, beliefs, practices, and institutions that regulate intimate relationships and that assume that adulthood involves stable commitment to a couple relationship. Some beliefs that support the couple-norm are the beliefs that a couple relationship will:

- Be approved of by the families of the two people involved
- Be homogamous (between people with similar economic and social backgrounds)
- Involve marriage and lifelong commitment
- Be based on romantic love
- Be sexually monogamous
- Involve work by both partners

Roseneil *et al.* contend that:

> As the extended family has tended to recede from daily life and the nuclear family has been losing its hold on individuals, intimate life choices have proliferated. Women's greater economic and social independence and the profound reshaping of cultural expectations and personal desires by feminist and lesbian and gay movements have foregrounded the ideals of equality, self-actualization and individual rights and freedom. This has contributed to the rising numbers of people who are living alone, remaining unmarried, divorcing, de-domesticating their sexual and love relationships, living openly with, marrying and divorcing same-sex partners. Yet… against the backdrop of these changes…the tenacity of the couple-norm comes sharply into focus (p. 3).

Erikson endorses the couple-norm by setting forth an intimate, committed emotional and sexual relationship as the prerequisite to becoming a healthy adult. Along with this, for Erikson, goes the ability to set boundaries to protect oneself from damaging relationships. Both intimacy and boundary-setting require a sense of identity for oneself vis-à-vis others. But there are many ways in which we can form empathic and supportive connections to others, with or without a couple relationship or a sexual component. A well-known instrument, the UCLA Loneliness Scale (Hughes *et al.*, 2004) is often used in surveys to measure how close and connected people feel to others. None of these indicators of connection and closeness depend on being in a couple relationship. Some examples of the indicators are:

- Feeling in tune with others
- Having companionship
- Having someone to turn to
- Feeling a part of a group of friends
- Feeling understood
- Having a lot in common with others
- Having people to talk to
- Sharing interests with others
- Feeling close to people

Erikson does not place as much emphasis on the establishment of an occupational commitment as he does on the development of intimacy, probably because of his Freudian background, which emphasizes psychosexual development. Still, he recognizes that this is also an important struggle in early adulthood. The struggle to establish oneself in an occupational role can be a difficult one, especially for those with who have not established a sense of identity, have less education, have qualifications that are not suited to labor market, or those in areas with high unemployment rates. The aspect of developmental arrest that most concerns parents of adult children in this stage in the U.S. is known in popular parlance as "**failure to launch**", referring to the fact that the adult child is not financially independent and has not established their own household or family. There is evidence that the percentage of American adults living in their parents' homes has increased markedly over time in the U.S. (South & Lei, 2015) and in other countries (Ronald & Alexy, 2011; Winsor, 2018). Winsor advocates for the addition of an intermediate stage called "emerging adulthood" to take into account this changing reality.

In Japan, there is concern about the growing problem of what has been labeled hikikomori, "a situation where a person without psychosis is withdrawn into his/her home for more than six months and does not participate in society such as attending school and/or work" (Saitō, 2012). Horiguchi (2014) reports data showing the presence of hikikomori-like cases in other countries, including Hong Kong, Oman, Spain, India, South Korea, and the U.S. He notes that there are still no evidence-based resources for the condition and posits that it is still a hidden epidemic in other countries. The internet plays a big role in the expanding hikikomori problem and Horiguchi anticipates that with further advances in Internet society, more and more people may come to live a hikikomori-like existence, which may or may not be seen as a pathological condition at that time. The coronavirus pandemic, which began at the end of 2019, increased unemployment and forced many people around the world into social isolation from which some may never emerge. Businesses and universities in Japan have come up with many resources that provide a semblance of intimacy to socially isolated individuals. They include robotic companions, social accompaniment services, customized digital texting boyfriends or girlfriends, temperature-sensitive digital hands to hold, and more (Egan, 2020). Except for some studies showing that religiosity is associated with authoritarian parenting and corporal punishment, there is little research on the relationship between spirituality and family functioning (Vermeer, 2014). Pryce & Walsh (2003), who believe that sharing transcendent beliefs and practices strengthens family functioning, also caution that marriage can bring up a number of spiritual and religious issues, including interfaith conflicts, beliefs about divorce and remarriage, and feelings about same sex unions. Family disapproval around such issues can affect a family for many years.

The second stage of adulthood in Erikson's scheme, **Generativity vs. Stagnation**, begins with parenthood and continues until retirement (another culture-bound concept, since not all economies offer retirement as an option). The central task of this period is to develop a sense of generativity, or an interest in establishing and guiding the next generation, typically through parenthood. For those who do not have children, generativity may still take the form of guiding, teaching, or mentoring the next generation or simply leaving a personal, professional, or creative legacy for the future. In some indigenous societies where parenthood is a prerequisite for leadership, options for the childless have included foster parenting or a form of ritual parenthood (Sangree, 1987). The challenge of generativity can also be framed as an issue of doing for oneself vs. doing for others with an eye toward the future, or "an orientation toward interpersonal and intergenerational connectedness as distinct from individuality" (Rubenstein *et al.*, 2015). Dollahite (1998) has argued that generative behavior is inherently spiritual because it "involves transcending selfishness, the demands of the present, and the attractions and distractions of one's own generation" (p. 469).

The Freudian term **narcissism**, which is greatly overused, has been applied to some of the personality traits that may result from an inadequate resolution of the task of generativity. These include a tendency to focus excessively on the self and ignore the needs of others. It is important to remember, however, that one need not actually be a parent to experience connectedness with others or concern for the future. Some longitudinal research has indicated that spirituality is positively related to what has been called healthy narcissism, or self-esteem and a positive sense of self-worth, and negatively related to the negative personality traits listed above (Wink *et al.*, 2005). Other research has found that a sense of spiritual superiority can alter the balance of this relationship. In studies conducted in the Netherlands, Vonk & Visser (2021) reported that scores on a spiritual superiority measure were more strongly related to narcissism than to self-esteem.

Kohlberg's next level of development, which he calls **Postconventional Morality**, has two stages, though, as previously mentioned, most adults do not reach this level. The first stage of Postconventional Morality is **Social Contract and Individual Rights**. Now that the individual can reason abstractly to resolve complex philosophical issues on their own, they may no longer be satisfied with simply taking on the attitudes of the influential. Instead, they use their own judgment to discern universal ethical principles such as non-violence or respect for human dignity. They see the relationship between the individual and society as a utilitarian social contract in which rules or laws exist to create the greatest good for the greatest number, even though they sometimes harm particular people. Fowler calls this level of spiritual development **Individual-Reflective Faith**, and it occurs when individuals begin to use their abstract reasoning abilities to question the beliefs with which they have been surrounded and become open to learning about other points of view. Through learning, questioning, and reasoning, they begin to construct their own belief system. Fowler's next stage, **Conjunctive Faith**, involves an even deeper kind of self-examination that involves questioning one's own strongly held and largely unconscious biases and prejudices that have accumulated due to one's social class, religious tradition, ethnic group, or membership in other social groups. Developing Conjunctive Faith permits one to hold on to one's truths while recognizing that they are "relative, partial, and inevitably distorting apprehensions of transcendent reality" (p. 198).

Kohlberg's final stage of moral development, reached by very few, he calls **Universal Principles**. People at this stage have developed their own moral standards, based on universal principles, and act on them even if it is against the law or results in disapproval or punishment. Fowler also refers to the universal in naming his final stage **Universalizing Faith** and, like Kohlberg, he acknowledges that this stage is very rare. Among the people he mentions as having reached this stage are Ghandi, Martin Luther King, Jr., and Mother Teresa. Other names that come to mind are the present Dalai Lama and Desmond Tutu of South Africa. Such people act courageously based on universal principles such as love or justice and are "contagious in the sense that they create zones of liberation from the social, political, economic, and ideological shackles we place and endure on human futurity" (p. 200). Hoare (2002), in a review that includes Erikson's unpublished writings, shows that

Erikson also had arrived at a vision of moral development that went beyond rigid adherence to ethical principles to an affirmation of universal principles. Ma (1988) has proposed a revised version of Kohlberg's last three stages for Chinese and other Confucian-based cultures:

- **Instead of Law and Order**, "Golden mean orientation and social system". This entails behaving in the way that most people in society would feel is right.
- **Instead of Individual-Reflective**, "Basic rights and relative rights". This perspective involves a distinction between the rights of society and the rights of the individual and a recognition of the rights or values that are specific to one's group.
- **Instead of Universal Principles**, "Universal ethical principles of natural harmony". In this stage people make decisions based on self-chosen universal principles that enable them to transcend conflicts between the individual and the majority.

Erikson's final adult stage was originally **Integrity vs. Despair**. In this stage, the earlier issues of trust vs. mistrust re-emerge at a much broader level and with a more obvious spiritual component. The issues become, does the individual trust the whole process of life and death? Is the universe seen as safe and trustworthy? Can the individual maintain hope in the face of aging and the prospect of death? The psychiatrist Robert Butler (1963) coined the term "**life review**" to refer to "the universal occurrence in older people of an inner experience or mental process of reviewing one's life." The process of life review supports a sense of wholeness and an acceptance that one's life had meaning and was worth living. Resolution of the earlier task of generativity also supports the development of ego integrity in older adults (Busch *et al.*, 2018). These authors also found in the same study, which was carried out in Germany, the Czech Republic, and Cameroon, that the development of a sense of ego identity reduced the fear of death. **Bearing witness**, or sharing, either orally or in writing, unjust and traumatic life events may promote ego integrity. Since psychological trauma is often caused by events that have historic significance, bearing witness may have profound effects on the awareness of those who experience the sharing. Jung emphasized the importance of integrating the "**shadow**" self in midlife and later years. For Jung, the shadow consists of the unconscious, unknown, or dark side of the psyche — dark because it consists primarily of socially unacceptable emotions and impulses that have been repressed in the process of socialization as the individual develops a socially acceptable conscious personality, or persona. Though repressed, the shadow side of personality can still shape behavior, often blindsiding oneself or others. The shadow also contains positive, life-giving elements and Jung felt that becoming aware of one's shadow side and integrating it into one's conscious personality was an important task in mid- and later life.

Social engagement is an important predictor of physical and mental health and life satisfaction at all ages and while, overall, the number of social relationships a person has tends to decline with age, the number of close friends typically remains stable. Social isolation of the elderly, however, is a growing global problem. In Japan, this is known as the "8050" problem — situations in which parents in their 80s support hikikomori children in their 50's (Yoshioka, 2020). Experts in Japan and other countries are concerned that as the parents of older social isolates die, these isolates will lack social support and adequate financial resources. A Japanese Cabinet Office survey investigating "acute social withdrawal" conducted in 2016 (Tajan *et al.*, 2017) found that over 1.5 million Japanese people between the ages of 15 and 64 suffered from this syndrome, with the majority being male. To the extent that an individual has not been able to develop ego integrity in their later years, they may experience depression, hopelessness, bitterness, and regret as well as a fear of death.

In many communities and societies, a great deal of respect is accorded to older adults. This is particularly true in pre-literate societies where elders carry knowledge and history, transmitting it orally and bearing witness to events of the past. Elders have a special role in religious affairs in a number of contemporary religions and often function as leaders in indigenous societies. In West African Tuareg tribes, post-menopausal women have a special status and are required to increase their participation in tribal affairs (Rasmussen, 2000), confirming the anthropologist Margaret Mead's notion of "menopausal zest". Croning, a modern Neopagan rite of passage that honors a woman's passage into elderhood (Manning, 2012), is growing in popularity in English-speaking countries, along with "Sage-ing", a gender-neutral New Age practice.

To summarize, some adults go beyond conventional perspectives on spirituality and right vs. wrong to develop a "postconventional" morality that is more concerned with spiritual and moral principles than with rules, regulations, and doctrine. Another potential development in this stage is concern about future generations and leaving a legacy for society or the planet.

5.6 Ninth Stage

After Erickson's stage theory had received wide acceptance, his wife, Joan, suggested the need for a ninth stage to describe processes that occur with the frailty of later old age as bodily functions begin to fail (Erikson & Erikson, 1998). This phase involves a positive kind of withdrawal from the world and its concerns, termed "disengagement" by Cumming & Henry (1961). The Eriksons used Tornstam's concept of "**gerotranscendence**" (1989), which implies spiritual growth because it is a "shift from a materialistic and rational view of the world to a more cosmic and transcendental one" (Wadensten, 2007). Some observable changes include (Tornstam, 2005): a decreased fear of death (though there may be apprehensiveness about the process), greater comfort with mystery and the unknown, increased ability to take pleasure in small things, a blurring together of past and present, and an increased frequency and intensity of childhood memories. Such a change in outlook, of course, can begin much earlier in life but, if it has not already begun, it is often precipitated by the challenges of diminishing ego and impending death. In 1969, Elisabeth Kübler-Ross, a pioneering psychiatrist who worked with the terminally ill, developed a stage model for death and dying that was based on interviews with dying people themselves (2011). She distinguished five stages in the process:

1. **Denial:** Disbelief and refusal to face reality
2. **Anger:** Recognition that death is impending and anger at oneself, others, and perhaps God for remembered or imagined acts of omission or commission
3. **Bargaining:** Creating an illusion of control by attempting, for example, to "beat the disease", promising a behavior change in exchange for survival, or offering to accept death if it can only be postponed until after some important event has taken place

4. **Depression:** A sense of hopelessness and despair
5. **Acceptance:** Acceptance of the reality of one's prognosis and preparing for death while cherishing memories and enjoying the small pleasures that are still available

In a later book, she used these same stages, with slight changes in their descriptions, to describe the course of grief and grieving (Kübler-Ross & Kessler, 2005). Kübler-Ross cautioned that these stages were no means invariant or necessarily linear, that people may cycle back and forth through the stages, and that the process does not necessarily end in acceptance. Despite this caveat, mental health professionals often attempt to enforce this model, making their clients feel that they should be going through changes that they are not experiencing. This can be frustrating for the professional and damaging to the client because it interrupts resilience and makes them feel as if they are doing something wrong.

The term "funerary practices" is used to denote the beliefs and practices used by a religion or culture to remember and honor the dead. Many spiritual or religious funerary practices are based on a belief in the afterlife and are designed to help and protect the deceased on their journey to the next world. The French founder of the discipline of sociology, Emile Durkheim, focused on the social function of funerals (1916), arguing that they comfort the bereaved and bring people together to enable them to repair the ruptures in social connections that have been caused by a death.

Table 5.1 summarizes Erikson's, Piaget's, Kohlberg's, and Fowler's stages.

5.7 A non-linear perspective on spiritual development

Wilber, who writes from a transpersonal perspective, has further developed the ideas contained in Lovejoy's seminal work titled *The Great Chain of Being: A Study of the History of an Idea*, first published in the 1930s. He has created a complex and comprehensive non-linear model of levels of spiritual development (Wilber, n.d.). Wilber's conceptualization is not a stage theory because the stages are not connected to age ranges, and it does not assume that the different levels are consecutive stages. Instead, a person may be at different levels at different times or at more than one level at once. It is a very useful model and shows how a number of major religions conceptualize these

Table 5.1. Stages in development.

Age	Psychosocial (Erikson)	Cognitive (Piaget)	Moral (Kohlberg)	Spiritual (Fowler)
Infancy	1. Trust vs. mistrust	Sensorimotor	Intuitive morality	0. Undifferentiated faith
Early Childhood	2. Autonomy vs. shame and doubt 3. Initiative vs. guilt	Preoperational	Preconventional morality 1. Obedience/ punishment 2. Instrumental relativist	1. Intuitive projective faith
Childhood	4. Industry vs. inferiority	Concrete operations	Conventional morality 3. Good boy/nice girl 4. Law and order	2. Mythic-literal faith
Adolescence	5. Identity vs. identity confusion	Formal operations	Postconventional morality 5. Contract/ individual rights 6. Universal principles	3. Synthetic-conventional faith
Adulthood	6. Intimacy vs. isolation 7. Generativity vs. stagnation			4. Individuative-reflective faith 5. Conjunctive faith 6. Universalizing faith
Later Adulthood	8. Ego integrity vs. despair 9. Gerotranscendence			

levels. There are five ascending levels in his model, each level including and transcending the previous level:

1. (A) Matter, as described by physics
2. (A+B) Life, as described by biology
3. (A+B+C) Mind, as described by psychology
4. (A+B+C+D) Soul, as described by theology
5. (A+B+C+D+E) Spirit, as described by mysticism

The purpose of this chapter has been to integrate theory and research findings concerning biological, psychosocial, cognitive, moral, and spiritual development to provide a framework for guiding the clinical work of mental health professionals. Secure attachment in infancy is the foundation for healthy development of basic trust. As children become more competent and independent, they also learn to regulate their behavior in such a way as to avoid reproof and punishment and later internalize the behavior standards of their parents and other significant adults to make them their own. These changes are facilitated by cognitive changes that begin with a simple interest in the consequences of one's actions and progress through an understanding of relationships between concrete events to an ability to reason abstractly and think hypothetically. From the standpoint of moral development, an exclusive concern with one's own needs typically expands to include understanding the needs of others and a sense that one's own well-being rests in conformity to social standards for behavior. Faith development is seen as depending on cognitive and affective development and begins with the child uncritically adopting their parents' faith, internalizing it, and later becoming sensitive to the faith expectations of their wider community. Late adolescence and adulthood are often characterized by committed relationships and concern for nurturing others and/or leaving a legacy of some kind. Individuals may expand their sense of morality to understand it as a social contract that defines certain rights and responsibilities for the well-being of the entire community. Or they may even go on to think of morality in terms of universal principles, such as non-violence or non-discrimination, that transcend human laws. From a faith perspective, some people go on to take personal responsibility for their beliefs rather than conforming to external standards, and beyond that, to incorporate views from other faith traditions or even to consider people of all faiths part of a universal community. Later old age often brings frailty and disability but can also be a time in which the individual withdraws from the social and material world to experience a more cosmic and transcendent one.

Readers are cautioned not to take these stages too literally or to expect their clients to demonstrate them. They are simply ways of arranging modes of thinking and feeling to better understand people of different ages. The "great chain of being" shows a non-linear way of conceptualizing spiritual development that recognizes that people are capable of functioning at different spiritual levels whatever their age.

Discussion questions

1. John was a 23-year-old man who lived with his parents and refused to be vaccinated against the coronavirus at a time when a new, more contagious version of the virus was becoming widespread. John's father, who had been vaccinated, urged him get a covid shot, arguing that it would protect vulnerable people who could not be vaccinated for health reasons or because they did not have access to the vaccine. John refused, arguing that, because of his age, he was at low risk for serious consequences from the virus while the long-range consequences of the vaccine were unknown. He emphasized his right to protect his own health and make his own decisions.

   a. According to Kohlberg's moral development stages, what stage of moral development do you think John was in?

   b. What stage do you think his father was in?

2. Maria is a 40-year-old member of an evangelical church that believes it is necessary to have a "born again" salvation experience in order to go to heaven. Members are expected to actively proselytize their family and friends. Maria has many arguments with her mother, a practicing Catholic, because she fears her mother will go to hell unless she is "saved". Her mother argues back that Pope Francis has stated that even people who do not believe in God will be forgiven their sins if they follow their conscience. Maria's mother, in turn, is very upset by Maria's religious beliefs because she considers them narrow and exclusionary. She wants Maria to share her worldview.

   a. Which of Fowler's stages of development characterizes Maria? Her mother?

   b. Can you think of any way the two women could accept each other's perspectives?

3. Abernethy & Lancia (1998) present the following case: Ms. Y is a middle-aged, divorced Caucasian Catholic. She was experiencing symptoms of depression and anxiety in response to feelings of inadequacy as an employee, daughter, and mother. She attributed these concerns to her upbringing as well as her Catholic background...Ms. Y experienced guilt when she pursued pleasurable activities and viewed God as a punitive and wrathful father who sought to deny pleasure. The first phase of

treatment focused on her depression and her feelings of anxiety. The therapist then consulted with a colleague who recommended a book written from a Catholic perspective that highlighted the grace and mercy of God. The therapist, in turn, recommended this book to the client. The client also made a plan to speak with her priest about her beliefs.

a. Which of Fowler's stages best describes Ms. Y's beliefs?

b. What changes in her religious perspective might you expect as a result of her psychotherapy?

Exercise

The following is a situation Kohlberg & Kramer (1969) used to study moral development.

In Europe, a woman was near death from a special kind of cancer. There was one drug that the doctors thought might save her. It was a form of radium that a druggist in the same town had recently discovered. The drug was expensive to make, but the druggist was charging ten times what the drug cost him to make. He paid $200 for the radium and charged $2,000 for a small dose of the drug. The sick woman's husband, Heinz, went to everyone he knew to borrow the money, but he could only get together about $1,000. He told the druggist that his wife was dying and asked him to sell it cheaper or let him pay later. But the druggist said: "No, I discovered the drug and I'm going to make money from it." So Heinz got desperate and broke into the man's store to steal the drug for his wife. Should the husband have done that?

Watch this video in which three children respond to the Heinz dilemma: https://www.youtube.com/watch?v=CjPfI4Xu2CU. Write a paragraph comparing their stages of moral development.

Resources

Piaget's Stages of Development: https://www.youtube.com/watch?v=TRF27F2bn-A

Erik Erikson's Nine Stages of Development: https://www.youtube.com/watch?v=CWSaFHlNxwc&t=19s

James Fowler's Stages of Faith Formation: https://www.youtube.com/watch?v=0Ivi Waa_QuM

Kohlberg's Theory of Moral Development: https://www.youtube.com/watch?v=qsldxMlFbas

Carol Gilligan's Theory of Moral Development: https://www.youtube.com/watch?v=HctzZwwueL4

Chapter 6

Spirituality and Mental Health

Milner *et al.* (2020) have pointed to a "**religiosity gap**" between mental health professionals and their clients in the value they place on spirituality and religion. They argue that this often leads to the needs of the mentally ill being neglected. In their book, *Handbook of Spirituality, Religion, and Mental Health*, Rosmarin & Koenig (2020) acknowledge that religion is not a popular concept among mental health professionals or researchers, and that mental health professionals are considerably less likely than the general public to have a religious affiliation. Still, they point out that increasing attention is being paid to the relationship between spirituality and mental health both in research and clinical practice. Studies carried out with different populations and in different countries have found a positive relationship between spirituality and psychological well-being or mental health (e.g., Bożek, Nowak, & Blukacz, 2020; Hodapp & Zwingmann, 2019; Pandya, 2018a; Petkari & Ortiz-Tallo, 2018; Vaingankar *et al.*, 2021; Zare *et al.*, 2019). Research findings on the positive relationship between mental health and spiritual and religious beliefs and practices have been convincing enough that the U.S. Substance Abuse and Mental Health Services Administration, the federal agency responsible for determining whether research evidence supports the use of various mental health and substance use clinical interventions, has included spirituality in its model of the eight important dimensions of wellness[1] (Substance Abuse and Mental Health Services Administration, n.d.). A number of mental health professional organizations also provide guidelines

---

[1] The other dimensions are: social, emotional, intellectual, physical, environmental, financial, and occupational.

for integrating knowledge about spirituality and religion into their clinical practice (e.g., Pargament, 2013; Verghese, 2008).

6.1 Complex relationships to mental illness

As far as mental illness is concerned, most studies find a negative relationship between spirituality and/or religiousness on the one hand, and depression or bipolar disorder on the other (Mosqueiro *et al.*, 2020). The relationship between spirituality and mental health issues is not the same across all diagnostic categories, however. Some relationships are more complex. Positive spiritual/religious thoughts and beliefs are negatively related to anxiety, but negative spiritual/religious thoughts and beliefs are positively related to anxiety (Rosmarin & Leidl, 2020). While, overall, spirituality and religiousness are positively related to positive relationships and family well-being, situations in which they could intensify distress (e.g., unwanted pregnancy, divorce, sexual orientation) have barely been studied (Mahoney *et al.*, 2020). Studies of psychosis produce mixed findings: religiosity may be higher in those with psychosis and may, in fact, be a risk factor for psychosis but, at the same time, spiritual/religious beliefs and practices may be a resource for positive coping with psychosis (Huguelet, 2020; Pargament & Lomax, 2013). Similarly, religiosity can be a risk factor for eating disorders but also can be a positive resource for coping with body dysmorphia (Richards *et al.*, 2020). Religiosity is generally negatively related to substance use (Connery & Devido, 2020) and gambling (Grubbs & Grant, 2020), but these relationships, too, are complex because Connery & Devido found that spiritual struggles could actually be positively related to substance abuse and Grubbs & Grant found that, among those who do gamble, religiosity is positively correlated to the severity of the gambling issues. As far as sexual behavior is concerned, Grubbs & Grant found that religiosity is positively correlated with conservative sexual behavior but also with compulsive sexual behavior.

As many of the above findings indicate, there can be considerable overlap between the spiritual issues and the mental health issues that clients bring to therapy. This is confirmed by the fact that the widely used Diagnostic and Statistical Manual published by the American Psychiatric Association since 1994 has included a diagnostic code for a "Religious or Spiritual Problem". This category is used when "the focus of clinical attention is a religious or spiritual problem". The examples given are "distressing experiences that involve loss or questioning of faith, problems associated with conversions to a new faith, or questioning of spiritual values that may not necessarily be related to an organized church or religious institution" (American Psychiatric Association, 2013b). Abramowitz & Buchholz (2020) have found, for example, that it may be difficult to distinguish obsessive-compulsive religious scrupulosity from healthy religious practices. Obsessive-compulsive features include degree of rigidity and extent of interference with normal functioning, but because some religions are more controlling than others, context must also be taken into account.

Kim-Prieto (2014b) has identified characteristics of religions that may affect their influence on psychological well-being. These are:

- The extent to which the religion is nurturing and supportive as opposed to restrictive and negativistic.
- The extent to which the religion is valued in the individual's culture.
- The extent to which the religion is internalized and intrinsically motivated as opposed to being externalized and extrinsically motivated (though this distinction is based on findings from research on Protestant Christians only).
- The extent to which the religion provides coping strategies and the types of coping strategies it provides.

6.2 Spirituality and mental illness

Pargament & Exline (2020) have reviewed the literature on the ways in which spirituality in general or religion in particular can also be a source of stress and struggle by arousing painful questions during difficult times. They report their own previous research showing that such struggles are reported by about 30% of the general population (Wilt *et al.*, 2016) and cite other studies showing that, among people being treated for a mood disorder, about 50% report spiritual or religious struggles (Murphy *et al.*, 2016; Rosmarin *et al.*, 2014). They group spiritual and religious struggles into three categories:

1. Supernatural struggles involving perceptions of deities or demonic/evil forces

2. Intrapsychic struggles that reflect strains and tensions about spiritual or religious beliefs, moral issues, and ultimate meaning, and
3. Interpersonal struggles that involve conflicts with other people about religious or spiritual issues

Taylor (2016) has drawn a distinction between mental health "breakdowns" or psychoses, and what he calls spiritual "shift-ups" or awakenings. He acknowledges that some researchers believe there is no fundamental difference between the two, since both consist of going beyond the boundaries of the normal self, which can become either a psychotic or a spiritual experience depending on different factors such as the individual's ego-strength and the extent to which the experience is supported or pathologized by the person's peers or culture. Taylor argues that a spiritual awakening is fundamentally different from psychosis in that it involves:

> A shift into a different, higher-functioning state in which a person's vision of the world and relationship to it are transformed, along with their subjective experience and sense of identity. This shift brings a sense of well-being, clarity and connection. The person develops a more intense awareness of the phenomenal world, and a broad, global outlook, with an all-embracing sense of empathy with the whole human race, and a much-reduced sense of group identity.

These sudden awakenings often occur in the context of trauma such as bereavement, loss, failure, or severe stress and can cause emotional distress and cognitive disorganization. They can be misdiagnosed as psychoses. In the course of his dissertation research, Taylor found four individuals with sudden spiritual awakenings who were seen by psychiatrists, given medication, and/ or confined to mental hospitals (*ibid*). Taylor argues that there is a fundamental difference between psychoses and what Grof & Grof (1986) call a "spiritual emergency". They offer the following indicators that an experience can be regarded a spiritual emergency rather than a psychotic break:

- Transcendental, mythological, or archetypal themes
- Absence of organic brain disorder
- Absence of a physical disease that could cause delirium
- The presence of an "observing self" that sees the experience as an inner psychological process

Both psychotic and spiritual crises involve altered states of consciousness. Because spiritual crises can involve confusion, hallucinations, and delusions while religious and spiritual delusions and hallucinations can occur in psychoses, it can be difficult to distinguish between the two possibilities. Loewenthal & Lewis (2011) suggest that psychotic experiences of visions, voices, and the like can be distinguished from non-psychotic religious ones because the psychotic experiences are generally more unpleasant, unwanted, and uncontrollable.

Kaselionyte & Gumley (2019) have reviewed the literature on "extreme mental states" associated with meditation and have found two different approaches suggesting two distinct types of therapeutic response: a biomedical approach, which sees them as mental illnesses, and a spiritual approach, which sees them as spiritual emergencies. They argue that, while the two approaches involve different therapeutic choices, there is no reason why they cannot be combined in particular situations. St. Arnaud & Cormier (2017) differentiate among four variations of distress involving religious or spiritual content:

1. Purely religious problem: concerns of faith and doctrinal matters that should be treated by appropriate clergy rather than mental health professionals.
2. Mental disorders that manifest religious or spiritual symptoms (for example, an individual with a psychotic disorder who believes they are Jesus Christ).
3. A religious or spiritual problem concurrent with a mental disorder (for example, a person with obsessive-compulsive disorder who engages in excessive religious rituals).
4. A religious or spiritual problem not attributable to a mental disorder. This would include distressing religious, spiritual, or transpersonal experiences not directly linked to or caused by a psychological disorder (such as near-death encounters, mystical experiences, or spiritual emergencies).

These authors emphasize the importance of determining an individual's prior functioning when assessing an individual with spiritual or religious symptoms. When there is a history of normal development, good pre-episode functioning, a stressful precipitating experience, and a positive, exploratory attitude toward the experience as meaningful or growth promoting, a diagnosis of spiritual emergency should be considered. The treatment of a spiritual emergency consists of providing safety and containment so that the individual can gradually integrate the experience into their identity and worldview. Kállai & Kéri (2020) have used an instrument known as the Bonn Scale for the Assessment of Basic Symptoms to compare individuals with religious/spiritual crises to those with psychosis and found that both groups scored high on items measuring perplexity, self-disorder (disturbance of self-awareness), depression, and anxiety, but only those with psychosis received high on items measuring disturbance of social contact and cognition.

Religious fundamentalism has a complicated relationship with mental health and mental illness. Altemeyer & Hunsberger (1992) define religious fundamentalism as:

> The belief that there is one set of religious teachings that clearly contains the fundamental, basic, intrinsic, essential, inerrant truth about humanity and deity; that this essential truth is fundamentally opposed by forces of evil which must be vigorously fought; that this truth must be followed today according to the fundamental, unchangeable practices of the past; and that those who believe and follow these fundamental teachings have a special relationship with the deity.

In the U.S., we tend to focus on Christian or Muslim fundamentalism, but religious fundamentalism is a perspective that can be found in many different religions. In Judaism, for example, militant religious Zionists, the Ashkenazim, and the Sephardim all stress the need for strict conformity to the sacred Jewish writings. Buddhist fundamentalism has become common in some Asian countries such as Sri Lanka and Myanmar. Hindu fundamentalism in India has been described as "religious nationalism" because the Hindu religion does not have texts specifically designated as sacred, but there is a nationalistic, or even tribal, component in most religious fundamentalist groups and belief systems. Liht *et al.* (2011) have conducted an extensive review of the literature and identified seven characteristics of fundamentalism that place it in opposition to modern secularism:

1. Belief in revealed traditions rather than rational criticism
2. Heteronomy (moral absolutism and authority) rather than autonomy and relativism

3. Traditionalism rather than religious change
4. Religious authority rather than secular authority in the public arena
5. Secular culture is perceived as a threat rather than embraced
6. Belief in the superiority of a particular religion rather than religious pluralism
7. "Millennial-Messianic imminence" versus prophetic skepticism

Some have argued that the fundamentalistic mindset is symptomatic of mental disorder. In 2012, the British neuroscientist Kathleen Taylor suggested that religious fundamentalism was a mental illness for which neurological causes would soon be found. Since then, research has found a connection between prefrontal lobe damage and religious fundamentalism (Zhong *et al.*, 2017). The prefrontal cortex is the area of the brain responsible for "cognitive flexibility" or the ability to switch from one concept to another and hold in mind multiple concepts at once. It is also connected to open-mindedness or the willingness to entertain new ideas. Unterrainer *et al.* (2016) found a positive relationship between spirituality and healthy personality except in the case of religious fundamentalism, which was positively related to personality disorders such as narcissism and psychopathy.

Stanford & McAlister (2008) surveyed self-identified mentally ill Christians and found that the churches to which many of them belonged had dismissed their psychiatric diagnoses. Based on a review of the literature on religious fundamentalism and attitudes toward psychotherapy, Peteet (2019) reports that both Muslim and Christian religious fundamentalists tend to stigmatize those with mental health problems and to be mistrustful of mental health professionals, preferring to seek religious rather than psychological help. He points out that much more work is needed to identify and study models for working with faith leaders, congregations, and religious clients to reduce stereotypes of mental health professionals and stigmatization of mental illness. A Baptist pastor in Harlem, Michael Waldron, Jr., has drawn attention to what some call "**religious trauma syndrome**" (Schiffman, 2019). This refers to what Waldron calls the "weaponizing of scripture" to condemn gay, lesbian, and transgender people, pregnant single women, and many behaviors considered sinful. Warlick, Lawrence, & Armstrong (2021) have found a curvilinear relationship between scores on a religious fundamentalism scale and anxiety in sexual and/or gender minority individuals, with anxiety being highest in those who scored very low and those who scored very high. Another concept that is relevant here is the "**spiritual bypassing**", a term coined by Wellwood (2000). It refers to the use of spiritual beliefs and practices to avoid the work of dealing with psychological issues or, as Wellwood put it, "to shore up a shaky sense of self, or to belittle basic needs, feelings, and developmental tasks".

This chapter has discussed findings and opinions concerning the positive, negative, and mixed effects of spirituality on mental health. While existing research does not come close to fully answering the many questions we have about the relationship between these two complex and multidimensional concepts, it suggests that the relationship between spirituality and mental health is primarily positive. Nonetheless, spiritual issues can produce psychological distress that becomes a clinical issue. The importance of distinguishing between spiritual struggles and mental health issues is discussed and mental health issues related to fundamentalist religious beliefs are described.

Discussion questions

1. For Sigmund Freud, spirituality was beside the point in mental health care. He viewed religion as infantile and God as a longing for a "father figure". For his contemporary, Carl Jung, spiritual growth was an essential part of mental health and psychotherapy was a process of profound spiritual development. How do you feel about Freud's and Jung's views of the relationship between religion and mental health? What is your view?

2. What spiritual issues were present for the client described below? What psychological issues? Did he qualify for a DSM-5 diagnosis? If so, which one? If not, why not?

In August 1986 I was 32, sober in AA for almost five years, and had worked the 12 Steps, but without much understanding of the spiritual dimensions of the program. I was an agnostic, leaning toward atheist. That summer my life began to fall apart — the details don't matter too much, except to say that my inability to let go of character defects was largely responsible, and my marriage was crumbling. I know I was psychologically suffering too: often in tears, alternately anxious and despairing, lots of bitter regrets at my own behavior. Finally, one night I went to visit a guy named Lou who I knew from AA. We sat on the porch of his rectory and I poured out all my troubles (which I'm sure he'd already heard a number of times in AA meetings). When I was done, he said, "Well, I don't really know what more I can say to you, though since I am a priest, I'd be glad to pray with you if you like." I said sure, feeling like what've I got to lose. He put his hand on my head and began to pray.

I can't remember the words, because something happened. It was like a bolt of lightning that started at the top of my head and went all the way down my spine. The starry night seemed immense. I began to cry. When Lou stopped praying I said, "What did you do to me?" He looked alarmed, and asked me what happened. I was unable to explain, but I think I said something about feeling God's presence. Lou became business-like. "OK, we have to baptize you," he said, and got the chrism and the holy water and, boom, I was a Christian.

I know how pompous or pious or just silly that sounds, but I don't know how else to say it. I had a heightened awareness of God and love everywhere I looked. My own problems became insignificant. My heart opened. The world seemed transformed. It was like being high on some great psychedelic drug that never let you down. Slowly it faded, but very slowly.

I felt changed, but I did wonder if this was healthy, if I was kidding myself somehow. Many of my friends were skeptical, and worried about me. I had a therapist I trusted a lot, and I went to him in the middle of this and said, basically, "OK, am I having a nervous breakdown? Because that's what a lot of my friends think." He replied, "Absolutely not. What you're describing is what people have described for thousands of years. You had a sudden experience of God's reality. In the East they call it "opening the third eye". In the West it's generally called "conversion", or a "road to Damascus" experience. But it sounds very real, and you don't sound the least bit mentally ill." That was a big relief.

Exercise

Watch the following video titled *Hard to Believe — A film about mental health and spirituality:* https://www.youtube.com/watch?v=Y9oubYAgZcU. Write a paragraph about your reaction to the video.

Resource

Spiritual experience or mental illness?: https://www.cbc.ca/radio/tapestry/rethinking-addiction-and-mental-illness-1.3472587/is-it-a-spiritual-experience-or-mental-illness-1.3472909

Chapter 7

Ethical Issues in Spiritual Competence

In a survey of over 2,000 members of the National Association of Social Workers (2001), it was found that most respondents dealt with spirituality in their clinical practices but they lacked sufficient ethical guidelines for decision-making in these situations and would have benefitted from more opportunities during their training to discuss the application of ethical standards to case examples.

7.1 Ethical standards

The ethical standards for mental health professionals are consistent with one another in many respects. Plante (2007) describes a set of ethical guidelines called the **RRICC Model of Ethics**, which is based on the ethical guidelines of the American Psychological Society but also draws on the ethical codes of other mental health professions in the U.S. and various countries. The letters in the acronym stand for: respect, responsibility, integrity, competence, and concern. The description of the model is modified below to be inclusive of the range of mental health professionals.

- **Respect:** Mental health professionals must respect the beliefs and values associated with a client's religion and for clients who seek religious and spiritual growth, development, and involvement, even if the professional does not agree with them. The clinician must also be respectful of the role that religious clergy and spiritual models have in the lives of spiritual and religious clients.

- **Responsibility:** Mental health professionals have a responsibility to be aware of and thoughtful about how religion and spiritual matters affect clients and to consult with and refer to religious and spiritual professionals as needed. When desired by clients, mental health professionals should work collaboratively with clergy and other religious leaders involved in their clients' care.

- **Integrity:** Mental health professionals must act with integrity by being "honest, just, and fair" with all those with whom they work. Integrity requires careful monitoring of personal and professional boundaries since they can easily become blurred when spirituality is integrated with psychotherapy. Unless they are also clergy and are explicitly acting as both mental health and clerical professionals, mental health clinicians must not act as experts in religious or spiritual areas that were not part of their professional training and licensure process.

- **Competence:** Mental health professionals must be aware of the limitations on their competence when they integrate spiritual and religious matters into their psychotherapy practice and be careful not to overstep their limits and skills. Whether or not they have received adequate instruction and supervision in their training programs, they must, on a continuing basis: keep up with the relevant literature, attend appropriate workshops and seminars, seek out consultation and supervision from appropriate colleagues, and learn more about the religious and spiritual traditions of the clients they typically encounter.

- **Concern:** While it is necessary to be respectful of those from various spiritual and religious traditions, religious and spiritual beliefs and practices can also cause harm to self or others. In those cases, the welfare of clients and others must be the mental health professional's paramount consideration.

Thus, when someone seeks to 'kill infidels", commit terrorism, or oppress and abuse others in the name of their religious tradition, our concern for others must force us to act to prevent harm. This concern might propel us to report child abuse, involuntarily commit someone to a psychiatric facility, or perhaps engage in other legal means to avoid any serious harm to self and others (Plante, 2007, p. 896).

7.2 Confidentiality

Client confidentiality is an issue when a mental health professional seeks clinician supervision or consultation with a cultural or spiritual authority. In these situations, the mental health professional must withhold any information that would enable the client to be identified. Clinical supervisors are ethically required to maintain the confidentiality of information about clients shared with them by the clinicians they supervise, but in other cases, the mental health professional must obtain written consent for the release of information from the client. Client confidentiality is often protected by the laws that apply in the jurisdiction where the mental health professional practices. In the U.S., the Health Insurance Portability and Accessibility Act regulates confidentiality at a national level (U.S. Department of Health and Human Services, n.d.).

7.3 Ethics and law

While mental health professionals in the U.S. are largely regulated through state boards consisting of members of their professions, there are also state and local laws that govern their practice. While most states have laws protecting client confidentiality in the therapeutic relationship, all permit and require the reporting of child abuse or neglect even though this is a violation of the principle of client confidentiality. Other countries with mandatory child abuse reporting include England, Ireland, Australia, Brazil, Denmark, Finland, France, Hungary, Israel, Malaysia, Mexico, Norway, South Africa, and Sweden. Research indicates that mandatory reporters in many countries have concerns about these requirements (Liu & Vaughn, 2019), including the risk of legal liability if they make an inaccurate report, damage to the therapeutic relationship, disturbance to family dynamics, and the risk of causing further harm to children. Clinical supervision should always be sought when deciding whether to report child abuse.

Another type of law in the U.S. that permits and requires breaching confidentiality is called "**duty to warn**". The duty to warn refers to a mental health professional's obligation to warn any identifiable potential victims when a client makes threats to harm them and has the means to carry out those threats. Duty-to-warn laws require the mental health professional to communicate to law enforcement and the intended victim in such a way as to protect the intended victim and protect them from being considered in violation of state laws protecting client confidentiality. The duty to warn also conflicts with the confidentiality requirements of the ethical codes of all mental health professions, so that a professional may have to choose between ethical code violations and breaking the law.

Other laws that it is important for the mental health professional to be aware of when including spiritual issues in their clinical practice have to do with licensure, because it is illegal to identify oneself as a member of a profession in which one is not licensed. For example, one may only claim to be a pastoral counselor if one is actually licensed by the state to practice that profession. Pastors without specialized training and licensure may offer pastoral care, but they cannot legally present themselves as pastoral counselors.

7.4 Client rights

Informed consent is another ethical requirement in psychotherapy. Clients have an ethical and legal right to be given all of the information about their proposed treatment that might reasonably be expected to influence their decision to participate in psychotherapy. The information should include other available treatment options and their risks and benefits. This includes information about the therapist's approach to spiritual issues if these are to be included in treatment. The American Psychiatric Association (2021) has issued a statement regarding the right of patients to receive services that their psychiatrist objects to, based on their own religious or spiritual principles. They state that such objections must never be permitted to compromise the quality, efficiency, or equitable delivery of medical services. Obviously, this is a situation that calls for supervision and perhaps consultation with a medical ethicist.

There is a great deal of variation among and within countries in whether and how the ethical codes and other guidelines of mental health professional associations define or require cultural competence. When cultural considerations are included in such documents, they may consist simply of an explicit non-discrimination statement, though the association may recognize the importance of a multicultural approach in some of the continuing education courses it offers for its members. For example, the Code of Ethics of the American Association for Marriage and Family Therapy (2015) stipulates that:

> Marriage and family therapists provide professional assistance to persons without discrimination on the basis of race, age, ethnicity, socioeconomic

states, disability, gender, health status, religion, national origin, sexual orientation, gender identity or relationship status.

Along the same lines, the Code of Ethics of the World Psychiatric Association (WPA) requires psychiatrists to "Respect patients' culture, ethnicity, language, and religion. They do not discriminate against patients on any grounds…neither do they attempt to impose their own values on patients and patients' families" (WPA Standing Committee on Ethics and Review, 2020).

Spiritual competence is often not mentioned in ethical codes though it is implicit in many of these statements. Some mental health codes are explicit about their guidelines for spiritual competence than others. For example, the American Counseling Association (2009) has issued a formal statement on competencies for addressing spiritual and religious issues in counseling based on their ethical code. The competencies are:

- Describing the similarities and differences between spirituality and religion, including the basic beliefs of various spiritual systems, major world religions, agnosticism, and atheism.
- Recognizing that the client's beliefs (or absence of beliefs) about spirituality and/or religion are central to his or her worldview and can influence psychological functioning.
- Actively exploring one's own attitudes, beliefs, and values about spiritual and/or religion.
- Continually evaluating the influence of one's own spiritual and/or religious beliefs and values on the client and the counseling process.
- Identifying the limits of one's own understanding of the client's spiritual and/or religious perspective and being acquainted with religious and spiritual resources and leaders who can be avenues for consultation and to whom the counselor can refer.
- Describing and applying various models of spiritual and/or religious development and their relationship to human development.
- Responding to client communications about spirituality and/or religion with acceptance and sensitivity.
- Using spiritual and/or religious concepts that are consistent with the client's spiritual and/or religious perspective and are acceptable to the client.

- Recognizing spiritual and/or religious themes in client communication and being able to address these with the client when they are therapeutically relevant.
- Striving to understand a client's spiritual and/or religious perspective by gathering information from the client and other sources.
- Recognizing, when making a diagnosis, that the client's spiritual and/or religious perspectives can a) enhance well-being; b) contribute to client problems; and/or exacerbate symptoms.
- Setting goals with the client that are consistent with the client's spiritual and/or religious perspective.
- Modifying therapeutic techniques to include a client's spiritual and/or religious perspectives and utilizing spiritual and/or religious practices as techniques when appropriate and acceptable to a client's viewpoint.
- Therapeutically applying theory and current research supporting the inclusion of a client's spiritual and/or religious perspectives and practices.

The American Psychiatric Association has prepared a Resource Document on Ethics at the Interface of Religion, Spirituality, and Psychiatric Practice (American Psychiatric Association, 2021) that states that psychiatrists should:

- Maintain respect for their patients' commitments (values, beliefs, and worldviews) by
  - Obtaining information on their religious/spiritual commitment.
  - Having empathy for their sensibilities and commitments.
  - Showing empathic respect when making interpretations that concern a patient's commitments.
- Not impose their own religious/spiritual, anti-religious/spiritual, or other values, beliefs, and worldviews on their patients, nor substitute such commitments or religious/spiritual rituals for professionally accepted diagnostic methods or therapeutic practice.
- Foster recovery by making treatment decisions with patients in ways that respect and take into meaningful consideration their cultural, religious, and spiritual ideals.

7.5 Spiritual competence

The term "spiritual competence" has not become as popular in other countries as it has in the English-speaking world, at least as yet, but concept of respect for the client's religious beliefs and practices is common to many ethical codes worldwide. Canda, Moon, & Kim (2017), for example, point out that it is common in Korea to address spirituality by referring to particular religions and that the Korean language does not have a word that corresponds to our word "spirituality". In their book, *Korean Social Welfare's Approach to Spiritual Diversity*, they actually had to coin a Korean term to talk about spirituality as distinct from religion. Whatever one's mental health profession, and whatever one's country of practice, it is essential to be aware of the appropriate ethical standards and guidelines and to seek consultation when in doubt as to how to apply them. The Association for Spiritual, Ethical, and Religious Values in Counseling (ASERVIC) has broken down the requirements for ethically addressing spiritual and religious issues in counseling into six categories. These requirements can be applied across mental health professions.

1. **Culture and worldview**
   The ability to describe similarities and differences between spirituality and religion and the basic beliefs of various spiritual systems, major world religions, agnosticism, and atheism.

2. **Counselor self-awareness**
   Active exploration of one's own attitudes, values, beliefs about spirituality and/or religion; continuous evaluation of the influence of one's beliefs and values on the client and the counseling process; and identification of the limits of one's own understanding of the client's religious and/or spiritual perspective and acquaintance with religious and spiritual resources, including leaders, with whom one can consult and to whom one can refer.

3. **Human and spiritual development**
   The ability to describe and apply various models of spiritual and/or religious development and their relationship to human development.

4. **Communication**
   Response to client communications about spirituality and/or religion with acceptance and sensitivity; use of spiritual and/or religious concepts

that are consistent with the client's spiritual and/or religious perspective and that are acceptable to the client; recognition of spiritual and/or religious themes in client communication and ability to address these with the client when they are therapeutically relevant.

5. **Assessment**
   During the intake and assessment processes, striving to understand a client's spiritual and/or religious perspective by gathering information from the client and other sources.

6. **Diagnosis and treatment**
   Understanding, when making a diagnosis, that a client's spiritual and/or religious perspectives can enhance well-being; contribute to client problems, and/or exacerbate problems; setting goals with the client that are consistent with the client's spiritual and/or religious beliefs; modifying therapeutic techniques to include the client's spiritual and/or religious perspectives; utilize spiritual and/or religious practices as techniques when appropriate and acceptable to a client; applying, therapeutically, theory and current research supporting the inclusion of a client's spiritual and/or religious beliefs and practices.

Hodge (2007) has developed an eight-item spiritual competence questionnaire and scale that can be used to assess social work programs. It contains the following questions (*ibid*, p. 290):

1. To what degree does your social work program foster respect for religious and spiritual cultures?
2. How acceptable is it in your social work program to share religious or spiritual views?
3. To what extent does your social work program foster sensitivity toward religious and spiritual beliefs?
4. To what extent does the atmosphere in your social work program foster respect for religious and spiritual perspectives?
5. To what degree are religious or spiritual believers free to be themselves in your social work program?
6. If spiritual or religious perspectives are shared in your social work program, to what extent are they valued?
7. To what extent does your social work program foster an empathic understanding of religious and spiritual worldviews?

8. When it comes to learning about the religious and spiritual worldviews that clients commonly affirm, how much openness does your program demonstrate?

Like the ASERVIC standards, these questions can be asked across mental health programs.

7.6 Ethical issues

Lomax *et al.* (2002) identify four levels of intervention that integrate psychotherapy and spirituality and caution each ascending level is more difficult to justify ethically than the preceding level. The first level is inquiry into the religious or spiritual beliefs, practices, and affiliations of the client. When tactfully managed and especially if prompted by a reference on the part of the client to a spiritual issue or affiliation, it is relatively easy to justify ethically as a normal part of ongoing client assessment. The second level is participation in a religious or spiritual activity with the client. This may include such activities as leading or joining in prayer (as long as the prayer concerns spiritual matters and is not a prayer for healing as a part of therapy) meditation, dispensing counsel or advice, encouraging the sharing of hopes, doubts and anxieties, or an offering of support and comfort. The ethical questions raised by these activities include the possibility of undue clinician influence due to client transference (client autonomy), and the scope of practice of the mental health professional (competence). Such ethical issues can often be resolved by referring the client to, consulting with, or collaborating with persons within the client's own spiritual or religious tradition. The third level is recommending that the patient participate in religious or spiritual activity for their well-being. The fourth is recommending that the client cease participating in a spiritual or religious activity for their well-being. The third and fourth levels raise ethical issues such as respect for client autonomy and provider competence as well as clinical issues such as transference and counter-transference. For the third and fourth levels, the authors suggest that the mental health professional share empirically based information with the client but refrain from making recommendations. This does not apply in cases of child abuse or neglect or a threat to the life of the client or others, in which case the clinician has an obligation to inform the appropriate authorities (see Section 7.5).

These authors also discuss three different scenarios. In the first, the clinician is negatively disposed toward religion and the client is a devout believer. If the clinician is unable to relate empathically to the client's beliefs, it may be necessary to refer the client to a different mental health professional. In the second scenario, the clinician is a fervent believer and feels called to draw others to their faith. In this case, the mental health professional is ethically obligated to share their "religious sensibilities" with the client. They suggest a statement such as:

> I can see that a number of issues are troubling you. Through our work together I hope to help you cope better with these challenges in your life. Because I happen to be a religious person, I will not only give you the benefit of my best efforts, but in my religious devotions, I will also be praying for a successful outcome to our efforts (*ibid*, p. 11).

If the communication is as limited as the one above and the client has a compatible faith orientation, there is no ethical problem though such a statement may influence the clinical course of treatment, especially in the areas of transference and countertransference. In the third scenario, the mental health professional is concerned that a client's religious or spiritual belief is harmful to their mental health. It may be that the client's interpretation of the relevant teaching is not correct. When this happens, the therapist might suggest, after consultation, that the patient discuss their interpretation with a spiritual or religious leader. If the consultation reveals that the client's belief is supported by their clergy or spiritual leader, it is ethically appropriate for the therapist to share their concern with the client but continue therapy with the client by mutual agreement or refer the client to another mental health professional.

In his description of the RRICC model, Plante discusses four "ethical pitfalls" that can emerge when spirituality is integrated into clinical practice. It is important to bear in mind that consultation and supervision must be used as needed to resolve ethical issues.

1. **Integrity issues: Blurred boundaries and dual relationships.** Licensed mental health professionals must report child abuse and neglect to the police or to child protective services. It is important that mental health professionals make this clear to their clients. For those who are both mental health professionals and clergy, it is especially important to

explain this mandate to clients. Another common ethical dilemma occurs when a mental health professional is an active member of a spiritual or religious group and receives referrals from their clergy. Since dual relationships are prohibited or discouraged in professional codes of ethics, depending on the type of relationship or circumstances, this can cause a dilemma for the mental health professional. Plante recommends taking into consideration the nature of the professional work, the size of the religious congregation, the type of possible dual relationships that might emerge, and the need for clarity of roles and responsibilities.

2. **Respect issues: Spiritual and religious bias.** It can be difficult for a mental health professional to overcome their own spiritual or religious biases when working with a client who has a different orientation, but this is required by their clinical licensure and professional ethical guidelines. Plante notes that ongoing consultation or supervision may be required.

3. **Competence issues: Being a member of a faith tradition does not make one an expert.** Mental health professionals must avoid acting in roles that are outside their area of competence and licensure such as pastoral care, spiritual direction, or theological consultation unless they have been professionally trained and certified in these areas. One must make one's areas of competence clear to clients and refer to other professionals, including members of the clergy, when necessary.

4. **Concern issues: Destructive beliefs and behaviors.** Religious convictions can lead to warfare and terrorism at the extreme and also in less destructive, but still harmful, behaviors. For example, members of some religious groups may refuse medical treatment for their children or believe that physical punishment of children and women is appropriate. Others practice female circumcision or deny females education. Respect for clients' religious beliefs does not require the mental health professional to be complicit in physical or mental harm, abuse, or neglect as defined by law or ethical codes. For example, even if a client justifies child abuse or neglect on religious grounds, the mental health professional is still required to break confidentiality and report the matter to authorities.

Transference and **countertransference** are important ethical considerations in all clinical encounters but are of special ethical concern when integrating spiritual approaches and tools into psychotherapy. A positive transference may cause a client to be overly accepting of a perceived point of view on the part of their therapist or to project the attitudes of other prominent figures in their life onto the therapist. A negative transference can also cause the client to misperceive their therapist's point of view. This means that the clinician must be attentive to the transference and support the client's autonomy. Mental health professionals must also be aware of their own countertransference issues as they affect their own reactions and attitudes toward clients. Abernethy & Lancia (1998) describe four kinds of "religiocultural" transference and countertransference:

1. Interreligious transference: the patient perceives that they and the therapist have different religious backgrounds.
2. Intrareligious transference: the patient perceives that they and the therapist have similar religious backgrounds.
3. Interreligious countertransference: the therapist perceives that they and the patient have different religious backgrounds.
4. Intrareligious countertransference: the therapist perceives that they and the patient have similar religious backgrounds.

They emphasize that transference and countertransference can occur in spiritually integrated psychotherapy not only when the patient and the therapist have different religious perspectives, but also when they share the same religion or even the same denomination.

Barnett & Johnson (2011) propose an eight-step ethical decision-making model for dealing with religious and spiritual issues in psychotherapy. The steps are:

1. Respectfully assess the client's religious or spiritual beliefs.
2. Carefully assess any connection between the presenting problem and religious or spiritual beliefs and commitments.
3. Weave the results of this assessment into the informed consent process. If processing religious or spiritual issues or experiences is needed for progress in psychotherapy, communicate this to the client, giving careful consideration to the client's level of insight concerning this need. Disclose any elements of your values and beliefs that might facilitate or seriously impede developing a positive therapeutic relationship. Obtain the client's consent to your treatment plan before implementing it.
4. Honestly consider your countertransference to the client's religiousness or spirituality. If it threatens to interfere with the therapeutic process or harm the client in any way, seek consultation and consider referral.

5. Honestly evaluate your competence in this case using prevailing standards of competence. Seek up-to-date information about the client's faith community.
6. Consult with experienced colleagues who have demonstrated competence in the relevant areas of spirituality, religion, and practice.

This chapter has described ethical standards common to mental health professions and discussed the kinds of ethical issues that are likely to arise when spiritual issues are addressed in clinical practice. The importance of understanding both the ethical standards of one's profession and the legal requirements concerning mandatory reporting, confidentiality requirements, and scope of practice is emphasized. Clinical supervision is essential in providing clinical and ethical guidance to mental health professionals around spiritual issues in psychotherapy and should always be sought when making difficult ethical decisions. In addition, consultation or even collaboration with spiritual leaders sharing the client's perspective is an important resource.

Discussion questions

1. Winslow & Wehtje-Winslow (2007) have argued that it is unethical for health care professionals "to prescribe spiritual practices or urge patients to relinquish religious beliefs or practices". Using the following case as an example, do you agree or disagree with them?

Ms. A is a single, 18-year-old, evangelical Christian who recently matriculated at a conservative Christian college. Ms. A. has a history of bipolar II disorder, which a psychiatrist in her home state has successfully managed for three years. During her previous treatment, the patient's religious beliefs were never an issue. She is now seeking advice from Dr. M, a psychiatrist who considers himself an agnostic, about whether she should continue taking a mood stabilizer. Ms. A. states, "I have done really well on lithium — in fact, that's how I made it to college. But now, I'm conflicted. My psychology professor — who is also an elder of the church I attend in town — is telling me that I should depend on the Lord, not on medication. He also says I would have been healed by now, if I had put my trust in God and not in a psychiatrist, who, he says, are mostly atheists. My mother said similar things to me when I first started on lithium, and she didn't want her church friends to know that I was seeing a psychiatrist. But I still don't feel comfortable stopping the medication, especially during my first semester of college, because I'm afraid that I will have mood swings again. On the other hand, am I going against God's will by remaining on lithium? What do you think, Dr. M?" (Pies & Geppert, 2013).

2. Consider the following dialogue between two social workers in a family counseling agency (Barsky, 2019). Consult the ethical guidelines of your mental health profession and think about how you would respond to Roger if you were Ella.

Roger: I've just conducted an intake interview with Mr. Perez. I'd like to refer him to you. I think it would be a better fit. [Note: Ella identifies as a lesbian.]

Ella: Thank you, Roger. I'm wondering why you think it would be better for Mr. Perez to work with me.

Roger: Mr. Perez says he is gay, which fits more with your area of expertise.

Ella: I certainly welcome working with clients of all sexual orientations. However, I would also hope that you could work with gay clients.

Roger: As you know, I am Christian, and homosexuality is viewed as an abomination in my religion. It's partly an issue of who can serve this client better, but also a question of religious freedom. I don't think I should be forced to support a homosexual lifestyle. This would violate my core beliefs. [Note: Roger identifies as an evangelist Christian.]

Ella: As a social worker, isn't respect for the dignity and worth of all people one of our core beliefs? Don't we have an obligation to provide service to all people, regardless of their sexual orientation?

Roger: Yes, respect for all is important, including respect for the religious beliefs of social workers. And yes, I do believe clients have a right to access to services, which is why I am referring Mr. Perez to you.

3. The Markkula Center at Santa Clara University describes a case in which confidentiality and duty to warn are in conflict (https://www.scu.edu/ ethics/focus-areas/bioethics/resources/confidentiality-and-duty-to- warn/). What are the ethical and legal considerations in this situation? (For a discussion of options, click on the link above.)

You are a psychologist treating a 22-year-old man with a history of depression and generalized anxiety who works in retail. He is despondent because he has learned a young woman, Susan, who works the counter with him, is dating another man. In the past he referred to Susan as his girlfriend. However, when you queried him about that he described her friendliness at work, not situations you would consider dating. He says her new relationship is "not right". He shares a fantasy of stalking Susan and her new boyfriend on a date and suddenly appearing in order to "catch" them and give them a "good scare". When you ask if he ever desires to hurt them, he says no, just to scare them.

Exercise

Look up a copy of the ethical standards and guidelines of your professional organization and write several paragraphs explaining what they say, either explicitly or implicitly, about spiritual competence. Below are links for many organizations. If yours is not listed below, conduct an internet search.

Resources

American Association of Marriage and Family Therapists — Code of Ethics: https://aamft.org/Legal_Ethics/Code_of_Ethics.aspx

American Counseling Association — Ethical and Professional Standards: https://www.counseling.org/knowledge-center/ethics

American Psychiatric Association — The Principles of Medical Ethics with Annotations Especially Applicable to Psychiatry: https://ajp.psychiatryonline.org/doi/abs/10.1176/ajp.130.9.1057?journalCode=ajp

American Psychological Association Ethical Principles and Code of Conduct: https://www.counseling.org/knowledge-center/ethics

National Association of Alcoholism and Drug Abuse Counselors — Code of Ethics: https://www.naadac.org/assets/2416/naadac_code_of_ethics_112021.pdf

National Association of Social Workers — Code of Ethics: https://www.socialworkers.org/About/Ethics/Code-of-Ethics/Code-of-Ethics-English

World Psychiatric Association — Code of Ethics: https://3ba346de-fde6-473f-b1da-536498661f9c.filesusr.com/ugd/842ec8_1d812c6b8a4f4d24878ee1db8a6376f6.pdf

European Psychiatric Association — Code of Ethics: https://www.europsy.net/app/uploads/2021/06/EPA-Code-of-Ethics_March-2021-GA-approved.pdf

International Union of Psychological Science — Universal Declaration of Ethical Principles for Psychologists: https://www.iupsys.net/about/governance/universal-declaration-of-ethical-principles-for-psychologists.html

International Federation of Social Workers — Global Social Work Statement of Ethical Principles: https://www.ifsw.org/global-social-work-statement-of-ethical-principles/

ASERVIC Competencies: https://www.counseling.org/docs/default-source/competencies/competencies-for-addressing-spiritual-and-religious-issues-in-counseling.pdf?sfvrsn=aad7c2c_10

Chapter 8

Assessing Spiritual Orientations, Needs, and Goals

A U.S. survey that included counselors, marriage and family therapists, social workers, psychiatric nurses, and psychologists found that while all of these professions held very positive attitudes about integrating spirituality into their therapeutic process, only about half of them included questions about spirituality in their assessment (Oxhandler & Parrish, 2017). Hodge (2015) offers six reasons why mental health professionals should conduct spiritual assessments of their clients:

1. **Compliance with professional codes of ethics**. Most ethical codes for mental health professions prohibit discrimination based on religion and require professionals to respect their client's religious orientation. Though respect for spirituality is often not explicitly mentioned, it is implied.
2. **Respect for clients' basic human rights**. The United Nations Universal Declaration of Human Rights (1948) prohibits religious discrimination and protects religious freedom, also implying spiritual freedom.
3. **Protecting client autonomy**. Client autonomy and self-determination is a central ethical principle which means that clients who want their spiritual values integrated into the clinical services they receive should have that option.
4. **Identification of strengths** that can be used for problem solving or to facilitate coping.
5. **Provision of culturally competent services.**

6. **Adherence to professional standards** for good practice as articulated by accrediting agencies and professional organizations.

Spiritual assessment need not be thought of as a separate component of the assessment process. There are many ways in which learning about a client's spiritual orientation, needs, and struggles can be integrated into the basic assessment process. Even before undertaking spiritual assessments of clients, however, and on an ongoing basis, clinicians should conduct their own spiritual self-assessments. Ideally, this process should begin in their graduate training. Dudley (2016) suggests that students in social work programs should be provided with opportunities to discuss their varied spiritual and religious beliefs with the intention of learning more about one another without any attempt to judge, influence, or control what others believe. This helps them learn about variations in religious and spiritual experiences but also helps them clarify their own attitudes and beliefs. Such discussions need not be limited to academic settings. We all have the opportunity in our daily lives to express interest in others' beliefs and practices and to listen without judgment while becoming aware of our own. Clinicians can also use the assessment tools described below, as well as others, to reveal and clarify their own attitudes and beliefs.

8.1 Strengths-based vs. medical approaches to assessment

Lee (2019) advocates a strength-based approach to spiritual assessment in which the clinician assesses the client's spiritual strengths in order to use them as resources in treatment or identifies spiritual struggles for which the client needs support. This can be contrasted to a medical approach that identifies and pathologizes mental disorders to create a treatment plan. Both approaches are clinically useful in assessment.

8.2 Opening the conversation

Scull (2015) uses the term "spiritual cues" to refer to client verbal and non-verbal communications that can create an opening for a therapist to show a willingness to discuss a client's spiritual concerns. Examples include concern about the client's own or someone else's death, expressions of faith, wearing clothing or jewelry that represents spiritual or religious beliefs, or expressions of guilt or remorse. If the client does not present an opening in early sessions, it is best to wait a few sessions to raise the question of spirituality in order to allow time for the establishment of rapport.

8.3 Brief spiritual assessments

There are a number of different commonly used approaches to carrying out a brief spiritual assessment, probably the simplest of which is known as **OPEN INVITE** (Saguil & Phelps, 2012):

1. **OPEN:** Open the door to conversation.
2. **INVITE:** Invite the patient to discuss spiritual needs.

Many of the approaches are known by acronyms that create mnemonic devices because they include the first letters of the key words.

The **FICA** questions (Pulchaski, 2006):

1. What is your **faith** or belief? Do you consider yourself spiritual or religious? What things do you believe give meaning to your life?
2. Is it **important** in your life? What influence does it have on how you take care of yourself? How have your beliefs influenced in your behavior during this illness? What role do your beliefs play in regaining your health?
3. Are you part of a spiritual or religious **community**? Is this of support to you and how? Is there a person or group of people you really love or who are really important to you?
4. How would you like me, your health care provider, to **address** these issues in your health care?

The **HOPE** questions (Anandarajah & Hight, 2001) were developed in a medical setting to provide information about the following:

1. Sources of **hope**, meaning, comfort, strength, peace, love, and connection
2. **Organized** religion
3. **Personal** spirituality and practice
4. **Effects** on medical and end-of-life decisions

The **iCARING** questions (Hodge, 2015) addressed these issues:

1. **Importance:** Importance of spirituality or religion
2. **Community:** Attendance at church or spiritual community
3. **Assets and resources:** Helpful spiritual beliefs and practices
4. **Influence:** Influence of spirituality on understanding of and response to present situation
5. **Needs:** Spiritual needs or concerns that could be addressed
6. **Goals:** Interest in incorporating spirituality into work and, if so, how that would look

The **MIMBRA** questions (Canda & Furman, 2010):

1. **Meaning:** What helps you experience a deep sense of meaning?
2. **Importance:** Are spirituality, religion, or faith important to you?
3. **Membership:** Are you a member of any groups or communities?
4. **Beliefs:** Please describe any important beliefs, practices…or values?
5. **Relevance:** (Is any of what we have discussed so far) relevant to your current situation and your goals?
6. **Action:** Are there close friends, relatives, mentors, clergy or spiritual teachers whom I should be aware of or contact?

8.4 Implicit spiritual assessment

An implicit spiritual assessment is one that does not mention spirituality, religion, or practices such as prayer or meditation that are associated with various religious traditions. Instead, they are humanistic or existential in their approach, asking questions about past, present, and future sources of joy, meaning, sense of hope, resources for coping with challenges, sources of vitality, insights, meaningful practices or other nourishing experiences (Canda & Furman, 2010; Hodge, 2015).

8.5 Spiritual history

A client's spiritual history can be obtained in an unstructured format or guided by a structured set of questions. They may or may not reflect chronology. Hodge (2015) notes that spiritual histories appeal to highly verbal people who enjoy face-to-face interaction and are congruent with cultures that value storytelling and/or oral transmission. Spiritual history-taking is client-centered and may help build a therapeutic alliance as well as being potentially therapeutic in themselves. The spiritual history need not be a separate process but can be integrated into ongoing clinical conversations as needed or indicated. Hodge & Holtrop (2008) have identified several questions that can be helpful in obtaining a spiritual history:

- Describe the religious/spiritual tradition you grew up in. How did your family express its spiritual beliefs? How important was spirituality to your family? Extended family?
- What sort of personal experiences (practices) stand out to you during your years at home? What made these experiences special? How have they informed your later life?
- How have you transitioned or matured from those experiences? How would you describe your current spiritual/religious orientation? Is your spirituality a personal strength? If so, how?

8.6 Graphic representations

A historical timeline is a graphic representation of events along a line in the order of their occurrence. A **spiritual timeline** is a historical timeline that shows a person's spiritual influences, insights, experiences, beliefs, practices, and changes over time (Figure 8.1). It can be helpful when taking a spiritual history. Curry (2009) points out that it is helpful to have a physical representation of a client's spiritual history that the client and therapist can refer to during therapy sessions. She notes that it is important to explain what a timeline is, ask for the client's consent, and provide appropriate materials such as white paper, construction paper, markers, and colored pencils. The client may wish to bring photographs or other memorabilia to add to the

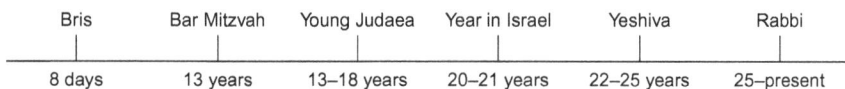

Bris	Bar Mitzvah	Young Judaea	Year in Israel	Yeshiva	Rabbi
8 days	13 years	13–18 years	20–21 years	22–25 years	25–present

Figure 8.1.   Sample of a spiritual timeline.

timeline. Hodge (2005a) also advocates the use of spiritual timelines, which he calls "spiritual lifemaps".

Spiritual ecomaps or ecograms can be used to assess an individual's, couple's, or family's relationship to various other spiritually relevant people, groups, and systems. They are used to portray relationships to spiritual traditions, communities, spiritual mentors and companions, transpersonal forces or entities, and faith leaders. The individual, couple, or family is shown as a large central circle surrounded by other circles to denote relationships (Figure 8.2). The surrounding circles are connected to the central circle by lines that are depicted in ways that indicate their nature (for example, cross-hatched or jagged lines for a conflictual relationship, dotted lines for a weak relationship, single solid lines for a solid connection, and double solid lines for a strong, positive connection (Hodge, 2000, 2005b). The figure below shows a spiritual ecomap for Diane, a woman from a conservative Christian family who fights with her constantly because of her involvement in a Buddhist sangha near her house. Diane is unsure of whether to continue this involvement because of the trouble it has caused in her family, but her husband, Robert, who considers himself neither spiritual nor religious, supports her affiliation with the sangha, as does his family, who are Ethical Humanists.

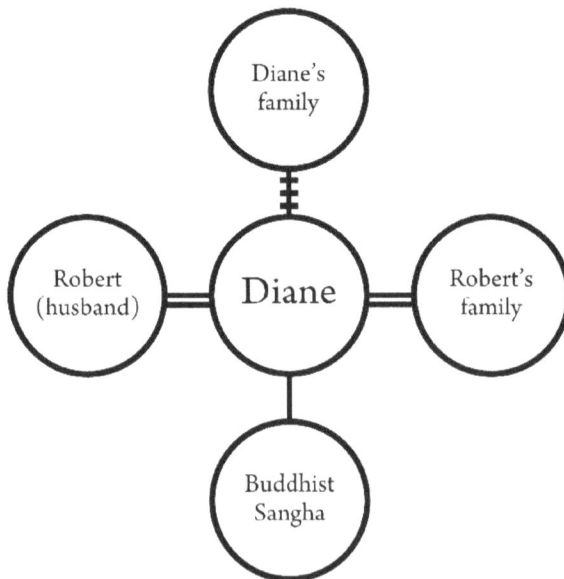

Figure 8.2.   Sample of a spiritual ecomap.

A genogram is a diagram that shows the relationship between a client, their family members, and their ancestors along with relevant information about each individual. A **spiritual genogram** shows information about spirituality and religious affiliations. Genograms are typically created by the clinician based on questions used to the client. Spiritual genograms can be helpful in understanding the family and cultural context of a client's spiritual beliefs and values. They can also be useful in highlighting spiritual strengths and resources within families and in identifying family conflicts. Hodge (2001) recommends including three generations in the genogram and, if relevant, other figures who have been significant in the client's spiritual history. The sample genogram below (Figure 8.3) portrays three generations of a family with both Hindu and Baptist religious ties. In a genogram, squares have traditionally been used for males and circles for females, but **gender-inclusive genogram symbols** are being introduced (e.g., Barsky, 2020). The person whose family is being depicted is called the **index person** and is surrounded by a double line. The X in the box for David's Hindu grandfather indicates that he is deceased. David, a 30-year-old college professor, is the index person in this genogram, and David's parents are both Baptists. His father was born in India and raised as a Hindu, but met his wife, an American-born Anglo-European Baptist, when he came to the U.S. for college. His wife, David's mother, was raised in India by Baptist missionaries but returned to the U.S., where they still live now, for college. David visited both sets of grandparents in India seven years ago, when his paternal grandfather was still alive, and was deeply impressed by their country, their culture, and

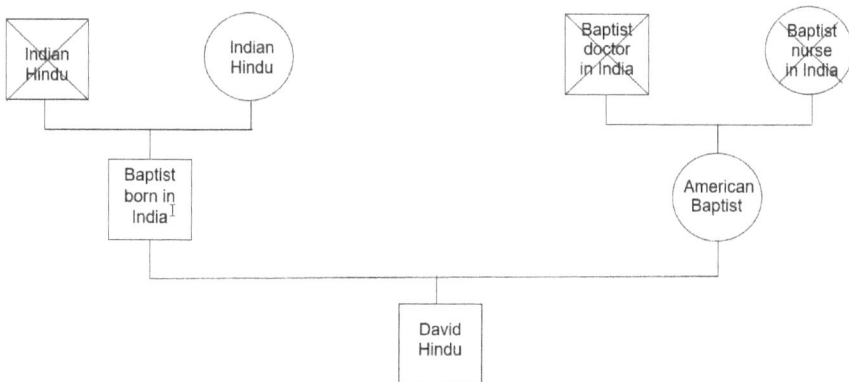

Figure 8.3.   Sample of a genogram.

their religion. Upon returning to the U.S., he began attending services at a local Vedanta center and engaging in the practices they taught. There is no formal conversion process in Hinduism, but he considers himself a convert and calls himself a Hindu. This has caused conflict with his parents, especially his mother, and he has become depressed and uncertain about his identity: Indian or American? His conflict with his parents seems to be aggravating his depression and identify conflict.

8.7 Spiritual issues and struggles

Dana (2018) has used polyvagal theory to develop a number of tools to assess clients' "**neuroception**". Neuroception is a term Porges (2011) uses to refer to the process by which neural networks determine whether situations or people are safe, dangerous, or life threatening. The relevant systems are the sympathetic nervous system (fight or flight) and the parasympathetic nervous system (ventral vagal, or connection, and dorsal vagal, or freeze). She provides three different formats for mapping the client's responses to safety and threat:

1. The **Personal Profile Map** helps the client and the therapist understand how the client's nervous system responds to danger and safety.
2. The **Triggers and Glimmers Map** helps the client identify triggers (provocations that are perceived as threatening) and glimmers (moments of safety and connection).
3. The **Regulating Resources Map** helps the client identify individual and interactive resources that aid them in building new regulating pathways.

These tools can be downloaded at: www.rhythmofregulation.com/Worksheets.php.

Vieten & Scammell (2015, pp. 61–62) define five areas of inquiry for the assessment of a client's spiritual struggles:

1. Exploring spiritual struggles
2. Exploring the extent of the client's struggle-related disorientation
3. Exploring the relationship of the spiritual struggles to the presenting problem
4. Exploring the client's past and present resources for coping with spiritual struggles
5. Exploring barriers to a resolution of spiritual struggles

Pargament & Saunders (2007) define spiritual struggles as "tension and conflict over matters of the sacred". Pargament & Exline (2020) identify five kinds of spiritual struggles:

1. Divine struggles: questions, conflicts, and tensions surrounding the individual's relationship to a deity or higher power. Struggles of ultimate meaning: the search for higher meaning or a sense of purpose in life
2. Struggles with doubt: the desire for truth and understanding
3. Moral struggles: the effort to resolve a moral conflict
4. Demonic struggles: struggles with demons or evil forces
5. Struggles with other people around spirituality or religion

Corbett (2011) distinguishes between depression and what has been called a "**dark night of the soul**" (taken from a poem written by the Catholic mystic and saint, John of the Cross, in the 1500s). While depression is a mental health condition, a dark night of the soul is a spiritual condition. Though it may have many of the same symptoms as depression, "a major concern of the person is that he or she feels spiritually impoverished or desolate, disconnected from the transpersonal realm, and is unable to pray or find meaning in his or her usual spiritual practices" (*ibid*, p. 121). In spite of this, the individual typically continues to remain effective in work and interpersonal relationships.

In this case, or in other divine struggles, this may be a circumstance in which collaborating with a clergy member or spiritual leader may be appropriate. Some clients may reject their faith over such a crisis while others may reach new understandings while remaining in their faith. It is important not to let one's own personal beliefs and biases influence the client's choices. Bayne & Tylsova (2019) encourage mental health professionals to be sensitive to the "God representations" of clients who believe in a higher being or power. They are concerned not just with the client's image of a deity, but also with the nature of their attachment to that figure, using attachment theory as a guide. They reference several assessment tools that are useful in measuring the attachment dimension of clients' God representations. In particular, they recommend Beck & McDonald's (2004) Attachment to God Inventory, which consists of 28 items that explore the degree of intimacy and/or distance between a client and their representation of God. It includes subscales that measure "avoidance of intimacy with God" and "anxiety about abandonment by God". The authors note that this inventory was constructed from a Judeo-Christian perspective and may need to be adjusted when working with other faiths or spiritual perspectives.

For Pargament & Saunders an **intrapersonal struggle** involves spirituality but takes place within the client. An example is being unable to forgive oneself for a transgression. Here, the role of the mental health professional is to include these issues in the clinical encounter just as would be the case for other intrapersonal issues raised by the client. Consultation with clergy from the client's church or the client's spiritual advisor may be helpful. An **interpersonal struggle**, such as feeling betrayed by a leader or member of one's religious or spiritual group or struggling with a family member over spiritual or religious beliefs, involves the client and another person. Helping clients work through these issues is an appropriate task for therapy.

Profound religious or spiritual experiences and insights can be disturbing and disorienting, causing a **spiritual crisis** with feelings and behaviors that resemble a mental health crisis (Vieten & Scammel, 2015). Some techniques to help people resolve a spiritual crisis include journaling, spending time in nature daily, engaging in regular exercise or movement, getting good nutrition and sleep, meeting with others who have had similar experiences, or carrying or displaying objects that remind them of the experience. Again, they recommend consulting with an expert if necessary. Several authors have described "red flags" or warning signs of **spiritual crisis** (e.g., Pargament & Brant, 1998; Mosqueiro *et al.*, 2020). They include:

- Self-neglect (devoting all of one's time to religion)
- Self-worship (turning away from spirituality and religion and focusing only on personal pleasure)
- Religious apathy (loss of sense of meaning, indifference to what happens)
- Fear or conviction of punishment by God
- Religious passivity (helplessness and failure to act due to total surrender to God)
- Religious vengeance (asking God to punish sinners)
- Religious denial (refusal to be upset by negative events because they are God's will)
- Interpersonal religious conflicts
- Anger at God
- Religious doubt

The DSM and the International Classification of Disease both now have a diagnostic category for a "religious or spiritual problem" that permits the differential diagnosis of spiritual problems and mental health problems. This category is described as follows in the DSM V:

> This category can be used when the focus of clinical attention is a religious or spiritual problem. Examples include distressing experiences that involve loss or questioning of faith, problems associated with conversion to a new faith, or questioning of spiritual values that may not necessarily be related to an organized church or religious institution (American Psychiatric Association, 2013b).

While the use of a V prefix for this condition in the DSM and a Z prefix in the ICD separate it from the diagnoses that indicate psychopathology, it also makes it unreimbursable by most health insurance plans, leaving the burden of payment for psychotherapy on the client who seeks care unless they have a comorbidity for which their insurance will pay.

8.8 Spiritual emergency or crisis vs. psychosis

Harris *et al.* (2020) describe a spiritual emergency as a process of spiritual awakening that becomes traumatic for an individual, leading to a state of psychological crisis, sometimes so severe that it resembles psychosis. Kaselionyte & Gumley (2019) have examined case reports of such "extreme mental states" and identified two very different styles of discourse. The first, which they call "biomedical", sees these experiences as psychiatric disorders while the second sees them as spiritual emergencies (Grof & Grof, 1986). In the former approach, therapeutic responses include hospitalization, restraint, psychiatric medication, and sometimes electroconvulsive therapy. Spiritual issues were typically not discussed. In the latter, they were conceptualized non-medically as cultural, spiritual, or psychological phenomena. Grof & Grof (1986) define spiritual emergencies as:

> Episodes of unusual experiences that involve changes in consciousness and in perceptual, emotional, cognitive, and psychosomatic functioning, in which there is a significant transpersonal emphasis in the process, such as dramatic death and (re)birth sequences, mythological and archetypal phenomena, past incarnation memories, out-of-body experiences, incidence of synchronicities or extrasensory perception, intense energetic phenomena (Kundalini awakening), states of mystical union, identification with cosmic consciousness (p. 1).

They argue that when these states are not the result of an organic brain disorder and when the client has not had a long history of conventional psychiatric treatment and hospitalization, a non-medical perspective should be applied to begin with. Spiritual emergencies, when managed properly, can result in spiritual emergence or spiritual growth.

8.9 Harmful beliefs and practices

Vieten & Scammell (2015) also discuss common types of harmful spiritually related beliefs and behaviors:

- **Negative religious coping:** Spirituality and religion can be very constructive in helping people cope positively with difficult experiences. Some frameworks that religions offer can result in negative coping (for example, blaming a child's illness on a punishing higher power). While negative coping may provide some relief by making sense of a situation, it has also been shown to be negatively related to various measures of mental health. These authors suggest asking a client who is using this type of coping whether this way of thinking makes them feel better or worse. It may just be a habit they grew up with rather than a central element in their current belief system.
- **Religious scrupulosity:** Scrupulosity is a feature of some obsessive-compulsive disorders and can involve an obsessive and overriding fear of having committed a sin or need to engage in compulsive behaviors to avoid divine punishment. Whether religious scrupulosity is caused by a mental disorder, religious beliefs, or both, the mental health professional should review the literature on religious scrupulosity and, if necessary, consult with an expert in the area.
- **Overinvolvement with spiritual and religious beliefs and practices:** While spiritual and religious beliefs and practices are correlated with better mental health, overinvolved clients perform them compulsively. Overinvolvement is indicated when it results in disturbances in functioning, disruption of relationships, avoidance of major responsibilities, extreme isolation, increased mental health symptoms, or physical pain or harm. It may be necessary to work with a clergy member, spiritual advisor, or teacher in the client's spiritual tradition to help the client find a more balanced level of involvement.

- **Belonging to a cult or cult-like group:** Cults are defined and viewed differently by different experts, as discussed in Chapter 2 of this book. Vieten & Scammell offer the following observations concerning cults. Defining a cult as "a group in which members hold a shared belief system that can go so far as to deny reality in order to sustain the social cohesiveness of the group", they caution that some spiritual groups have highly stylized rituals, tightly knit communities, and engage in unusual or unfamiliar activities without being cults. The key is not so much the content of what the group practices as it is the impact it is having on a client's well-being. They advise against directly confronting the client and instead recommend exploring the client's views non-judgmentally to learn more about how they became involved with the group and how it affects them. Signs that a spiritual or religious group may be harmful include the following:
    - The group has a charismatic leader who is controlling and considered beyond reproach.
    - The group requires excessive devotion or dedication to a person or idea.
    - The group requires its members to recruit others.
    - The group actively isolates members from family and friends.
    - Members are threatened psychologically or physically if they leave or consider leaving.

Working with clients on cult-related issues may be beyond the competency of most mental health professionals and require supervision, consultation, or even collaborating with an expert in this area.

8.10 Spiritually related abuse

The National Working Group on Child Abuse Linked to Faith or Belief in the United Kingdom has listed several spiritual beliefs that can lead to the abuse of children (2012). Included are a belief in:

- Witchcraft and spirit possession, demons, or the devil acting through children or leading them astray (traditionally seen in some Christian groups)

- The evil eye or djinns (traditionally seen in some Islamic faith contexts)
- Dakini (in a Hindu context)
- Ritual or "muti" (murder to obtain body parts for magical remedies) murders
- Use of belief in magic or witchcraft to create fear in children or make them more compliant

Though mental health professionals need to be aware of these possibilities, they caution that only a small minority of people with the beliefs listed above go on to abuse children. It is important not to stereotype or jump to conclusions. Other kinds of child abuse that can occur in a spiritual or religious contexts include excessively harsh discipline, physical and emotional abuse, pedophilia, and female genital mutilation. Spiritually related abuse is not confined to children. Enroth (1992) has described five ways in which adults can be abused by spiritual or faith-based groups:

1. Authority and power without openness or accountability
2. The use of fear, guilt, or threats to produce unquestioning obedience
3. Elitism and isolation from other groups and organizations
4. Insistence on rigid conformity in lifestyle and beliefs
5. Suppression of any kind of internal challenge to decisions made by leaders

Other types of abuse include psychological manipulation and financial and/or sexual exploitation. Leaving a spiritually abusing group can be difficult and traumatic. Winell (2006) coined the term "religious trauma syndrome" to designate the anxiety, depression, and other mental health issues that may be experienced by those who have left such a group.

This chapter has presented the reasons for conducting a spiritual assessment and techniques for doing it. Spiritual assessment is not treated as a one-time procedure to be carried out at the beginning of a therapeutic relationship but rather as an ongoing sensitivity to a client's beliefs, values, and practices and their actual or potential effects on the client's psychological well-being. Spiritual issues and struggles are described and the distinction between spiritual emergencies or crises and psychoses is considered. The mental health professional must also be alert to harmful spiritual beliefs and spiritually related abuse and seek supervision and/or consultation as needed.

Discussion questions

1. A "get" is a Jewish divorce that frees the former partner to remarry. Starr (2017) presents the following case:

    When Hannah Goldberg first met her husband, Daniel, he was friendly and charming. After a whirlwind courtship, they married and welcomed a son together. However, Daniel became increasingly critical of Hannah, and over time his behavior escalated into physical violence. When their son turned five, Hannah made the difficult decision to leave her marriage. The civil divorce process dragged out over several years, as the couple's son became the epicenter of a vicious custody battle. Finally, four years after she left her abusive husband, Hannah was a "free" woman under American law. However, she still did not have her Jewish divorce, or get, which would allow her to remarry under the laws of her Orthodox Jewish community. Hannah endured countless meetings with rabbis and religious courts and tried numerous times to offer Daniel money and other concessions in exchange for a get, to no avail (p. 37).

    Is this an example of spiritual abuse? Why or why not? If there is abuse, what role does the religious community play in it?

2. Park *et al.* (2017) present the case of a young woman who, in her first week of college, attended a fraternity party to welcome first-year students:

    She was given punch that had been laced with hypnotics and was subsequently sexually assaulted. Having grown up in a secure community and environment, it had never occurred to her that anyone would deliberately harm her; she felt betrayed by her college community and by God. She felt that she had been doing everything she could to do what she thought was right and interpreted the predestination beliefs of her church to mean that God had planned for this assault to happen to her. Her faith was severely challenged, and her acute trauma reaction was sufficiently disabling that she left college midway through her first semester, certain that she would not return to the same college, if she returned to school at all.

If she were your client, what questions would you want to ask her about her spiritual history, beliefs and/or practices?

3. Alberto is a 45-year-old schoolteacher whose husband, Martin, also a schoolteacher, has convinced him that he needs to seek psychotherapy. Shortly after his mother died, about six months ago, Alberto began having a series of profound mystical experiences in which his body seemed to dissolve and melt into what he called "the mystical wholeness of being". He would feel a profound sense of safety, peace and wholeness that was in stark contrast to the violence and destruction he saw in the everyday world. Martin is convinced that Alberto is mentally ill and Alberto does not know whether or not to believe him.

    If you were the psychotherapist in this situation, how would you go about assessing Alberto's mental health status?

Exercise

Conduct an internet search to determine what resources are available in your area for someone experiencing spiritual abuse. Write several paragraphs about what you found.

Resources

How to create a genogram: https://www.therapistaid.com/therapy-guide/genograms

This TED talk about indigenous cultures is entitled "Psychosis or Spiritual Awakening?": https://www.youtube.com/watch?v=CFtsHf1lVI4

The Attachment to God Inventory is useful for exploring secure, anxious, and avoidant relationships to a higher power: http://www.callisto-science.org/conference/Papers/ATTACHMENT%20TO%20GOD-THE%20ATTACHMENT%20TO%20GOD%20INVENTORY%20(McDonald,%20A.).pdf

The Spiritual Crisis Network in the UK provides peer support groups and email support for people who are undergoing a spiritual crisis: https://spiritualcrisis-network.uk/

The International Spiritual Emergency Network is in the process of creating links among spiritual emergence centers worldwide and assisting in the process of creating new networks where they do not yet exist: https://www.spiritualemergencenetwork.org/isen/

Chapter 9

Spiritually Competent Treatment

Saunders *et al.* (2010) have ordered approaches to integrating spirituality with mental health treatment along what they call a "continuum of spiritual care in psychotherapy" as shown in Figure 9.1. One extreme is characterized by outright avoidance of spiritual issues and topics (spiritually avoidant care) on the part of the mental health professional, which is inconsistent with culturally competent practice. At the opposite extreme (spiritually directive care), therapy focuses on a client's spiritual and religious beliefs and practices as "an explicit object of attention". This may be appropriate when these beliefs and practices relate to the resolution of the client's psychological problems but often may require the therapist to seek supervision and/or consultation. In spiritually directive care, the therapist may actually encourage the client to adopt certain beliefs and practices, raising ethical questions concerning competence, client autonomy, boundaries, and respect. Saunders *et al.* recommend, at a minimum, engaging in spiritually conscious care. This involves assessing a client's spiritual and religious practices and beliefs in a respectful and sensitive manner to determine their general importance to a client and their influence, if any, on the presenting symptoms and their availability as a resource for recovery. Spiritually integrated psychotherapy uses a

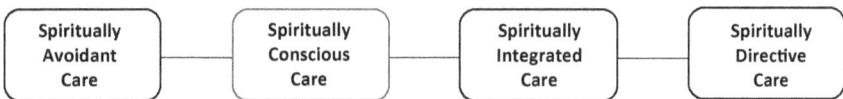

Figure 9.1. Continuum of spiritual care in psychotherapy. Source: Saunders & Miller (2010).

client's own spiritual and religious beliefs and practices to facilitate the goals of psychotherapy and sometimes may also use generic or ecumenical concepts as in the case of the concept of "higher power" in 12-step-oriented substance abuse treatment. Both spiritually conscious and spiritually integrated care must be used with caution because of the ethical issues described in Chapter 6 and because of the potential clinical effects of transference and countertransference. Spiritually directive care can involve recommending spiritual resources or activities but must be used with caution because of the issue of countertransference and competence. The greatest level of caution must be used when discouraging a spiritually related activity and should not be undertaken without supervision and/or consultation.

9.1 Jungian analytic psychology

There are a number of different models that offer guidance regarding the integration of spirituality and psychotherapy. In 1913, **Carl Jung** (1972) broke from Freud's biologically based psychoanalytic approach which saw the unconscious as a repository of infantile needs and fantasies. Instead, Jung emphasized the motivating power of spiritual needs and the importance of the unconscious as "a kind of infinite area within man, a spaceless space… more primal, more archaic, more primordial still than materiality" (Progoff, 1973, p. 166). This is the part of the inner self that mystics have traditionally referred to as the "ground of being" (Huxley, 1945) or the "seat of the soul" (Zukav, 1989). Jung used the term "collective unconscious" for that part of the unconscious that is present in all humans as a result of universally shared genetic predispositions, neurological processes, and developmental experiences. Archetypes are recurrent figures or symbolic patterns in the collective unconscious. The "shadow" is an archetype that consists of the aspects of self that are repressed because they conflict with the person the individual feels they should be. The shadow often appears in dreams as a frightening figure. Another archetype is the animus (for women) or the anima (for men). These consist of repressed feelings and traits attributed to the other sex and appear in dreams in various positive and negative forms.

Individuation is a central concept in Jung's approach and refers to the process of integrating the unconscious aspects of self with the persona, or the social face that one presents to the world, in order to achieve wholeness and find meaning in one's life. Jung felt that the analysis of dreams was an important strategy for revealing unconscious archetypes and integrating them with the conscious self. Another way of achieving wholeness through integrating the persona and the unconscious is to use what Jung called "active imagination", a state that bridges the gap between conscious and unconscious processes. It is evident in dreams, fantasies, creative expression, improvization, and symbols and often occurs during periods of transition between sleeping and waking. In fact, Julia Cameron, the author of *The Artist's Way* (1992), recommends keeping a notepad by the bed and making notes immediately upon waking in order to capitalize on the creativity of this interstitial space. The subtitle of her book is "A Spiritual Path to Higher Creativity".

Free association is another way of exploring the unconscious. In free association thoughts are allowed to suggest other thoughts in a flow of associations that lack any apparent connection but that are actually connected in the unconscious. Analysis of this "stream of consciousness" provides clues to unconscious processes (James, 1890). Another technique Jung used to encourage the use of active imagination was mandala drawing. A mandala is a symmetrical circular design containing concentric geometric shapes or symbols, considered in some religions to be a map of the universe and often used in these religions for ritualistic purposes. For Jung, it was considered to be a projection of unconscious aspects of the self. Fincher's (2010) guide is one of several books that describe methods for creating and interpreting mandalas.

A Jungian archetype that is especially relevant to the mental health professional's role in healing is that of the **Wounded Healer**. Victor *et al.* (2021) found that 82% of applied psychology graduate students and faculty members in the U.S. and Canada experienced mental health conditions at some point in their lives. Corbett (2011) writes at some length about the Wounded Healer in his book, *The Sacred Cauldron: Psychotherapy as a Spiritual Practice*. He says:

> The vocation to become a therapist has various sources. It partly results from developmental factors, such as the childhood need to care for an emotionally wounded parent…Often, the therapist-to-be has to become a therapist because his or her childhood wounding initiates him or her into a career of helping others. When the Wounded Healer archetype is dominant in the soul, one's own suffering enables one to help others. Our wounds affect the way we work with others, and the way we work with others affects our own wounds. Without one's own wound, one's understanding of the suffering of others would be superficial (p. 177).

Corbett points out that while woundedness can enhance a therapist's empathy and compassion, it can also raise countertransferential issues, including the possibility that the therapist may project their own wound onto the client or not be fully present to the client because the client's issue triggers their own pain. The enormity of the client's wound may cause the therapist to experience a compulsive need to help rather than support the client in finding their own solution, possibly resulting in burnout or despair. It is always important to seek supervision and/or therapy for oneself in these cases. Because Corbett views psychotherapy as a spiritual practice for the therapist, he also recommends the following practice when painful feelings are aroused by the countertransference:

> As long as the therapist can tolerate the painful affect, there is no need to resist it — to do so usually makes things worse. Instead, one can allow oneself to suffer with the person by connecting with the emotion that has been induced in one's body and focusing on it, as if the body were a sounding board. When projective identification occurs, the traditional advice is to pass the experience through one's own psychological structures and say something that will help the person "metabolize" and assimilate the emotion. This is not always done verbally; without saying anything, one can open the heart and allow the emotion to move as it will in the body. Usually, having risen to a crescendo, the distress gradually dissipates (p. 180).

9.2 The 12-step model

The 12-step model mentioned earlier (Ragins, 2006) originated in the self-help approach of Alcoholics Anonymous (AA), first described in a book with that title by its founder (Wilson, 1939). The 12-step program consists of regular peer-support meetings without professional leadership. The goal of these groups is abstinence from the problem behavior. Bill Wilson was influenced by Jung's views on spirituality and saw the 12-step program of AA as a spiritual solution to the problem of alcoholism. The original 12 steps of AA are (*ibid*):

1. We admitted we were powerless over alcohol — that our lives had become unmanageable.
2. Came to believe that a power greater than ourselves could restore us to sanity.

3. Made a decision to turn our will and our lives over to the care of God *as we understood Him.*
4. Made a searching and fearless moral inventory of ourselves.
5. Admitted to God, to ourselves, and to another human being the exact nature of our wrongs.
6. Were entirely ready to have God remove all these defects of character.
7. Humbly asked Him to remove our shortcomings.
8. Made a list of all persons we had harmed, and became willing to make amends to them all.
9. Made direct amends to such people wherever possible, except when to do so would injure them or others.
10. Continued to take personal inventory, and when we were wrong, promptly admitted it.
11. Sought through prayer and meditation improve our conscious contact with God *as we understood Him*, praying only for knowledge of His will for us and the power to carry that out.
12. Having had a spiritual awakening as the result of these steps, we tried to carry this message to alcoholics, and to practice these principles in all our affairs.

These steps are used for many different kinds of problems with modifications appropriate to the problem they target. For example, in Emotions Anonymous, a program for people with mental health issues, the first step is: "We admitted we were powerless over our emotions — that our lives had become unmanageable." Some other 12-step programs are AlAnon (for friends and family members of alcoholics), Overeaters Anonymous, Gamblers Anonymous, Debtors Anonymous, Sex and Love Addicts Anonymous, and Workaholics Anonymous. The steps also may be modified to eliminate the masculine pronoun for God, using "they" instead. The first three steps are often called the "surrender" steps because they involve admitting one has a problem and surrendering to a "higher power". The next six steps are referred to as the "housecleaning" steps because they address shame and guilt by requiring an honest self-appraisal and restorative actions. The last three steps are called the "maintenance" steps and reflect the AA principle that ongoing housecleaning, spiritual practice, and service to others are the best way to prevent relapse. Important tools in 12-step programs include:

- Attending 12-step meetings
- "Working" the steps with a sponsor
- Being of service in the program
- Prayer and meditation
- Celebrating anniversaries of "sobriety"
- Having a list of people to call when needed
- "Bibliotherapy", or reading recovery-oriented literature
- Practicing gratitude
- Practicing acceptance and surrender

A popular prayer in 12-step programs is the Serenity Prayer:

God, grant me the serenity to accept the things I cannot change, the courage to change the things I can, and the wisdom to know the difference.

Though 12-step programs are explicitly spiritual and use the terminology of the Abrahamic religions, they are not religious organizations, nor do they require any particular spiritual or religious beliefs. They are welcoming to both agnostics and atheists.

9.3 Motivational interviewing

Clarke *et al.* (2013) recommend a technique called motivational interviewing both for overcoming spiritual bypass and for supporting spiritual growth. Motivational interviewing is an evidence-based method of communication that encourages change. It originated in addiction treatment but is now used in many settings. It is especially useful when clients are ambivalent about change or lack confidence that they can change. There are four fundamental processes in motivational interviewing, though they are often circular rather than linear. They are:

- Building rapport through careful listening
- Negotiating agreement on a shared purpose or goal
- Evoking client's reasons and motivation for change
- Supporting a commitment to change and building a plan if the client is ready

The primary principles of this method are:

- Express empathy
- Roll with resistance — don't confront resistance directly, instead validate the client's right to make their own decisions and reframe their point of view or suggest other possibilities
- Develop discrepancy — help the client identify the costs and benefits of changing and not changing
- Support self-efficacy

Clarke and his colleagues describe a client who entered therapy with the goal of resolving a spiritual struggle with forgiveness around childhood sexual abuse. Through empathic listening the therapist was able to increase the client's awareness of her psychological issues and support her sense of a discrepancy within her religious beliefs that was hampering her psychological growth. The therapist also affirmed her self-efficacy, which permitted her to resolve both her psychological and spiritual struggles.

9.4 The Recovery Model

A model for mental illness that is similar to the 12-step programs has been called the **Recovery Model** (Walker, 2006). Like the 12-step programs, it views recovery as a process rather than a final outcome (members of 12-step programs, for example, typically refer to themselves as "recovering" rather than "recovered"). It is often used for the treatment of chronic or relapsing mental illnesses that can be managed but not entirely eliminated. The Recovery Model has been important in the design of community mental health programs in the U.S. and other countries, and it is of special value in developing countries with fewer mental health resources (Jacob, 2015). Its goal is to enhance the affected individual's functioning, increase their self-efficacy, and alleviate emotional distress. Jacob notes that the Recovery Model:

> …does not necessarily imply a return to premorbid level of functioning and asymptomatic phase of the person's life. Nor does it suggest a linear progression to recovery but one which may happen in "fits and starts" and, like life, have many ups and downs (p. 118).

In the Recovery Model, relationships between clients and mental health professionals are collaborative and frequently used tools include community mental health centers, drop-in centers, peer support groups, peer advocacy, and employment programs.

Lukoff (2007a; 2007b) and others have argued that spirituality should be an important dimension of the Recovery Model, just as it is in the 12-step programs. Lukoff contrasts what he calls the "recovery model" to the standard medical model of mental illness. Rather than trying to make a distinction between mental illness and spiritual crisis, Lukoff sees recovery from both as a spiritual journey, citing a body of research showing a positive relationship between spirituality on the one hand, and recovery from substance abuse and mental disorders on the other. He gives the following suggestions for spiritual support in recovery:

- Portraying recovery as a spiritual journey with a positive outcome
- Encouraging the client's involvement with a spiritual path or religious community
- Encouraging the client to seek support from reputable religious or spiritual leaders
- Encouraging the client to engage in religious and spiritual practices consistent with their beliefs
- Modeling one's own spirituality (when appropriate), including a sense of purpose and meaning, along with hope and faith in something transcendent

While the medical model tends to define recovery in negative terms (elimination of symptoms of psychopathology), the recovery model emphasizes recovery as described in the 12-step model that originated in the program of Alcoholics Anonymous. The recovery model as defined by Ragins (2006) involves:

- Accepting having a chronic, incurable disorder, that is a permanent part of them, without guilt or shame, without fault or blame.
- Avoiding complications of the condition (e.g., by staying sober).
- Participating in an ongoing support system both as a recipient and a provider.

- Changing many aspects of one's life including emotions, interpersonal relationships, and spirituality both to accommodate one's disorder and grow through overcoming it.

9.5 Existential and humanistic approaches

The Existential Model and the Humanistic Model refer to a broad range of different secular approaches to spirituality that emerged during the first half of the 20th century. The Existential Model emphasizes the universal human desire to find meaning and purpose in life. The Humanistic Model was popularized by Abraham Maslow and developed into what is now called "person-centered psychotherapy" by Carl Rogers. Both focus on the full development of the person's inner or "true" self, including its spiritual or transcendent aspects. (See Chapter 1 for a fuller discussion of Maslow's theory.) Rogers' major tool was what he called "unconditional positive regard", or expressing complete and authentic acceptance of a person without placing any conditions on this acceptance (1951). This validated the person's true self. Rogers was an agnostic, but as he got older, he also spoke about transcendental or mystical experiences, including the fact that the relationship between a client and a therapist capable of unconditional positive regard was, in itself, a spiritual experience (Thorne, 2002).

9.6 The Transpersonal Approach

The Transpersonal Approach, which also is used to refer to a variety of different holistic theories and treatment models, is defined by its emphasis on transcendent, spiritual, or transpersonal aspects of experience. Transpersonal psychotherapists may draw on any of a number of different techniques including journaling, mindfulness, meditation, guided imagery, breathwork, dreamwork, art, music, or hypnotherapy. Grof & Grof (1986) have discussed **spiritual crises** from a transpersonal perspective. They argue that though spiritual crises can resemble psychotic episodes, they are not the same thing, and the application of a medical perspective to a spiritual crisis, particularly the use of antipsychotic medications, can block the spiritual growth that such a crisis makes possible. Therapeutic approaches include support from a spiritual guide or teacher, "grounding" techniques, changing the diet, normalizing the experience, and temporarily refraining from spiritual practice. They recommend collaboration between mental health professionals and spiritual teachers and the use of a range of therapeutic approaches including both biomedical and alternative healing techniques. They caution, however, that it is important to monitor the effectiveness of the transpersonal interventions and be open to biomedical interventions if necessary.

Crowley (2006) has listed eight interventions, adapted from Lukoff (1998), that can be useful when working with clients struggling with a spiritual crisis:

1. **Normalization:** Crowley recounts Jung's (1964) intervention with a man in the midst of a spiritual crisis:

   I vividly recall the case of a professor who had a sudden vision and thought he was insane. He came to see me in a state of complete panic. I simply took a 400-year-old book from the shelf and showed him an old woodcut depicting his very vision. 'There's no reason for you to believe that you're insane,' I said to him. 'They knew about your vision 400 years ago.'

2. **Grounding:** Grounding consists of connecting the individual to their natural surroundings. Activities such as gentle exercise, walking outdoors, or gardening and a diet rich in "heavy" foods such as whole grain and beans is recommended, as well as dairy products and meat if the client's dietary restrictions permit. Sugar, caffeine, alcohol, and fasting should be avoided.

3. **Reduction of environmental and interpersonal stimulation:** The everyday world may be experienced as painful and interfering with inner processing. The therapist can help the client identify and avoid the specific people and situations that exacerbate the crisis. Crowley observes that "the sanctuary of a retreat center is ideal, an environment often in stark contrast to a psychiatric ward".

4. **Temporary discontinuation of spiritual practices:** Meditation, in particular, triggers many spiritual emergencies. Practices can be re-introduced once the person is more stable.

5. **Encouragement of expressive therapies:** Art, music, writing, poetry, dance.

6. **Creation of a therapeutic encounter:** Crowley recommends transpersonal psychotherapy or another spiritually integrated psychotherapeutic approach.

7. **Consideration for specific bodywork:** Bodywork refers to a range of therapeutic techniques, usually involving physical touch, that aid in healing. Examples are massage, acupuncture, and chiropractic. These therapies can help the person integrate the spiritual experience in a holistic way.

8. **Evaluation for medication:** While some believe that medication should not be used in spiritual emergencies because it can impede the person from their inner work, Crowley argues that when the crisis is so intense and anxiety-producing that the person is overwhelmed, it may be helpful to consider low doses of anti-anxiety or anti-psychotic medications to slow down the process and reduce the client's distress, allowing them to better assimilate the experience.

9.7 Faith-based models

Faith-based models incorporate the beliefs and practices of a particular religion into the psychotherapeutic process. Such a model may be appropriate when a client's religion is an important part of their life or when their religious community views psychotherapy with mistrust. Shared religious beliefs can be helpful in establishing and maintaining rapport with clients and the religion itself may provide helpful resources for coping. It is important that clinicians remember, however, that even if they share the client's religious beliefs, pastoral counseling is not a legitimate area of practice for them unless they are also credentialed in that discipline.

9.7.1 *Christian*

Most faith-based approaches are Christian, examples of which are most commonly found in English-speaking and some European countries. A collection of writings by an international group of Christian mental health professionals, the European Movement for Christian Anthropology, Psychology, and Psychotherapy, has been assembled by Joubert (2018). Joubert distinguishes between Christian psychotherapy models that use standard, empirically based interventions to achieve specific aims that reflect both clinical and spiritual objectives and those "charismatic" or "biblical" approaches that rely on "God's direct intervention through prayer". Empirically based clinical approaches that also incorporate Christian beliefs and practices reflect a variety of clinical and theological orientations and use a diversity of clinical and spiritual tools. Blanton (2019), for example, advocates the use of Christian contemplative prayer in counseling. Moodley & West (2005) call charismatic, or biblical, approaches "spirit-filled" because they attribute successful outcomes to God or the "Holy Spirit" rather than to the clinical process itself. Pfeifer (2007) presents a case history that illustrates how distinguishing psychosis from a spiritual breakthrough may be especially difficult when the therapist shares the client's religious beliefs. He tells the story of a young woman who became severely depressed and suicidal following her failure at a music academy and her father's sudden death:

> In therapy, she described her longing for heaven: "This life is but a preparation for eternal glory: there I will meet my father, there I will be able to praise God with my music which did not find the world's approval…" The patient's description of the promise of heaven…was so convincing that the therapist had to distance herself from that hope which she basically shared but which became dysfunctional in supporting suicide as the option to find the eternal bliss which the harsh reality of this world could not offer her.

9.7.2 *Jewish*

There is significant overlap between Christian and Jewish models because they both draw on the Hebrew scriptures, or what Christians often refer to as the "Old Testament", but they reflect different beliefs and practices as well as differences in cultural heritage. Rabinowitz (2010) uses the term "Judaic Spiritual Psychotherapy" to refer to a faith-based clinical approach that draws on the Hebrew scriptures and other Jewish teachings to counteract depression, hopelessness, and unrealistic guilt. He advocates the use of Jewish meditative practices and the practice of repentance (teshuva). He also recommends the practice of forgiveness (of oneself as well as others) but only when the offender has completed certain steps that, he notes, Judaism shares with other religious traditions. The offender must:

1. Take personal responsibility for the behavior
2. Express sincere regret
3. Make suitable reparation if possible
4. Promise to stop the offending behavior
5. Request forgiveness

These steps are necessary, he asserts, because without them, the extent of the client's injury is not acknowledged, and the client is rendered powerless.

9.7.3 *Islamic*

Carle (2018) observes that many practicing Muslims consider psychotherapy to be a Western science that is a threat to Islam. They strongly stigmatize the use of mental health services as a sign of weakness and lack of faith, believing instead that Quranic recitation and prayer are the solution to emotional problems. Islamic integrated approaches to psychotherapy can often make psychotherapy more accessible to Muslims. Keskínoğlu & Ekşí (2019) describe elements of Islam that can be used in counseling Islamic clients. They include:

- Praying together in sessions
- "Spiritual bibliotherapy", or using quotes from spiritual texts
- Reading the parables of the Quran
- Holding up religious role models from Islam and other religions
- Encouraging patience, submission to the will of God, gratitude, penitence, forgiveness of self and others, and contemplation
- Guiding clients toward the use of hymns that have a positive effect on mental health

They warn, however, that from an ethical point of view, the therapist must refrain from spiritual interventions that are not relevant to the psychological problem or the therapeutic objectives. When working with Muslim clients, it is important to be sensitive to their cultural and spiritual values. Though Muslims as a faith group include differing ethnicities and cultures, the mental health professional must be sensitive to how their beliefs affect their health care behaviors and preferences. Attum *et al.* (2021) list diet, ideas of modesty, touch restriction, and alcohol intake prohibition as important areas to be aware of.

9.7.4 *Hindu*

According to Mukherjee (2002), Hindu psychotherapeutic approaches see the chief cause of emotional distress as being ignorance. Two other major blocks are desire and karma, or the accumulated results of past actions in this life or previous lives. The antidotes to ignorance are truth, non-violence, and self-restraint. Hindu psychotherapeutic models stress non-dualistic thinking and the unity of all humanity, all experience, and all reality. Mukherjee lists four options for spiritual enhancement:

1. Abstract mental activities such as identification with the abstract principle of God, dedication of action to a Supreme Spirit, renunciation of "doership", or the sense that we are the doer of our actions, and of the "fruits of our actions"
2. Concrete ritual activities such as worship of a deity, following a spiritual leader, acting without a desire for results, and performing actions based on principles and verbally dedicating them to God
3. Emotional devotional actions such as becoming a devotee and worshipping, reducing other attachments, and viewing all beings as sacred
4. Practical simple daily actions such as singing hymns, chanting, meeting one's social responsibilities, non-violence, truthfulness, equanimity, and giving to the needy

9.7.5 *Taoist*

Tao is a Chinese word that means the way, or the path. Hagen (2002) uses the words "experiential" and 'intuitive' to describe Taoism. Intuition appears spontaneously as a result of experiential learning and formal study. Mindful living in the present moment is the goal of Taoism. According to Hagen, "Taoist mindfulness is silent, non-verbal, non-conceptual, and non-intellectual." Yin (darkness, the feminine, yielding) and yang (light, masculine, strong) are elements of the dialectical principle that underlies Taoism. The energy of all life is called "Chi". Internal imbalance of these elements or excesses/deficiencies of Chi cause poor health and distress. Meditation is an important tool in Taoism and Taoist psychotherapy and has four levels:

1. Centering the mind involves creating times of solitude in which the mind is quieted and ego defenses are gently relaxed
2. Emptying the mind of negative thoughts once it is centered
3. Grounding the mind once it is empty, cultivating intuition, imagination, and intellect
4. Connecting the mind and heart to experience unity, insight, creativity, and compassion for self and others

Hagen identifies a variety of other therapeutic strategies, including focusing-oriented psychotherapy, reflective listening, creativity, and attachment exercises, yoga, tai chi, and cognitive behavioral, gestalt, existential, or experiential therapies.

9.7.6 *Buddhist*

Buddhism is an outgrowth of Hinduism and both influenced and were influenced by Taoism. There are a number of Buddhist models for psychotherapy. Instead of viewing self-improvement as a goal, they tend to focus on developing compassion and love for ourselves and others. Olson (2002) identifies six principles that characterize many modern Buddhist psychotherapeutic approaches:

1. Acceptance of our emotions
2. Adoption of a "right view" in which we do not label or categorize our experience
3. Focus on the "here and now", meaning that we do not get caught up by memories or echoes from past experiences
4. Belief that body and mind are a single whole, not two separate systems
5. Appreciation of the importance of the environment, both the therapist's and the client's
6. Emphasis on the sanity that underlies all mental disorders

Morita therapy, developed by the Japanese psychiatrist Shoma Morita, is one of the earliest Asian therapeutic models that has gained a foothold in the U.S., especially since the 1970s, when it was popularized by David Reynolds (1976). Morita therapy is based in the nontheistic Zen philosophy and does not require that the client embrace Buddhism. Distressing feelings such as anxiety are seen as natural results of an individual's personality and their situation. Its goal is not to change disturbing feelings but rather to help the client accept the reality of the situation and whatever feelings are being experienced so that they can engage in positive behavior. The objective is not to eliminate the feelings but rather to help the person take constructive action in the present. Work is an important part of the therapy. Mruk & Hartzell (2003) identify six Buddhist principles in Zen psychotherapies:

1. Acceptance of suffering rather than denial
2. Courage in facing our fears
3. Choosing truth over illusion
4. Compassion toward self and others
5. Letting go of attachments
6. Accepting impermanence

Meditation is considered a useful tool for realizing these principles. Helderman (2019) has studied the approaches of psychotherapists who integrate Buddhist principles into their approach and finds that there is a great deal of diversity in how they apply these principles, depending on their clinical and spiritual training. Buddhist psychotherapy has also been called "contemplative psychotherapy" because of its emphasis on meditation but for most who apply Buddhist principles in their psychotherapy practice, it also involves an emphasis on compassion. Both are ways of freeing oneself from attachments and transcending ego. Acceptance and Commitment Therapy (ACT) is a Buddhist-influenced cognitive approach. Hayes & Smith (2005) have developed a comprehensive guide to exercises and practices that can be used by clients and mental health professionals. Nieuwsma *et al.* (2016) suggest that ACT can serve as a useful bridge for clergy to collaborate with mental health professionals. There is also a Christian version of ACT (Knabb, 2016).

Nguyen (2018) describes a daily 45-minute Buddhism-based group psychotherapy intervention that has been used in a mental hospital in Vietnam. It consists of meditation and meditation instructions, soothing music, relaxation exercises, and teachings from a Buddhist monk on such topics as kindness, compassion, the power of giving, or the law of cause and effect. After the session, clients do body stretching and breathing exercises. The clients reported that these sessions were useful but did not consider them a replacement for the medication they were receiving.

9.8 Ecospiritual approaches

Fisher (2011) has proposed what he calls a "**four domains model**" of spiritual health and well-being. The four domains are:

1. Personal, including meaning, purpose, and values
2. Communal, including morality, culture, and religion

3. Environmental, including care, nurture, and stewardship of the physical, eco-political, and social environment and connectedness to nature.
4. Transcendent, including Tillich's concept of "ultimate concern", the New Age concept of cosmic force, faith, and God for theists.

Ecospiritual approaches to mental health stress the environmental aspect of spiritual competence and spiritual health, stressing the importance of connection to and care for the Earth. Ecopsychology is an approach that integrates ecology and psychology and focuses on studying the emotional bond between humans and the Earth. The term "ecopsychology" was popularized by Theodore Roszak and first used in his book, *The Voice of the Earth*, in 1992. It refers to the connection between mental health and the health of the planet. The goal of ecopsychology is to awaken people to the "synergistic interplay between planetary and personal well-being" (Roszak & Gomes, 1995).

Ecopsychotherapy is a form of psychotherapy that is based on the principles of ecopsychology (Summers & Vivian, 2018). They describe such ecotherapeutic interventions as nature walks and "greencare". Greencare includes the therapeutic use of farming practices, animal-assisted interventions, social and therapeutic horticulture, and physical exercise undertaken in natural environments. There are now a number of graduate training programs in ecopsychology for mental health professionals, including certificate programs. Naor & Mayseless (2019) have identified four themes in clients' descriptions of their reactions to nature-based interventions:

1. Nature as an embodiment of the spiritual
2. The immensity of the natural environment as a stimulus to expand one's personal perspective
3. Interconnectedness with nature involves the experience of deeply belonging
4. Nature reflects inner aspects, provides unconditional acceptance, and inspires self-discovery

Rust (2020) defines ecopsychotherapy as follows:

Ecopsychotherapy is a relatively new form of psychotherapy which understands that human relationships exist within the larger context of life on earth. The web of life is not just a collection of beings but more like a continuum of earth–water–sky–tree–air–creatures–sun–human. Trauma arises when relationships within that continuum are disrupted; healing ourselves cannot be done in isolation. Psychotherapy invites us to tell the story of our human relationships; ecopsychotherapy expands this to include our earth story, the context or continuum in which our human relationships sit.

She suggests that a simple way of practicing ecopsychotherapy is to hold therapy sessions in a natural setting outdoors. Naor & Mayseless (2020) advocate "nature-based therapy", suggesting that it provides an opportunity to experience nature as an embodiment of spirituality, elicits a sense of interconnectedness and belonging to the "vast web of life", and contributes to the discovery of an "authentic self". Forest bathing (shinrin-yoku) is a traditional Japanese practice that involves visiting a forest, observing it, and breathing its air. Research shows that forest bathing reduces stress hormones (Antonelli *et al.*, 2019).

9.9 African-centered approaches

The continent of Africa is home to many different religions and spiritual perspectives and colonialism has had profound effects on indigenous beliefs. Bruchhausen (2018) has shown how the Western dichotomization of religion and medicine has secularized medicine in East African countries and regulated traditional healing practices according to Western "biomedical standards of safety and efficiency". Still, much of the indigenous approach to mental health and illness persists and can be integrated into psychotherapeutic processes. The traditional African worldview is a holistic one that attributes mental illness to a disruption of communal and spiritual ties, including ties to ancestral and other spirits. Graham (2005) lists three principal components:

1. The spiritual nature of human beings
2. The interconnectedness of all things
3. Oneness of mind, body, and spirit

Graham defines spirituality as "the creative life force, the very essence of all things that connect human beings to each other. Spirituality connects all elements of the universe — people, animals, and inanimate objects are seen as interconnected" (p. 213). Graham refers to the principle of Maat as an underlying guide for a harmonious relationship to the universe. The word Maat derives from an ancient Egyptian goddess who represents virtues such as truth, balance, harmony, propriety, and order as standards for living a good life. It is also seen as a kind of divine energy that flows through and sustains the universe. Bojuwoye (2005) notes that:

> The traditional African worldview makes no distinction between living and nonliving, natural and supernatural, material and immaterial, conscious and unconscious. Instead, these sets of phenomena are understood as unities (p. 62).

Communal living, called "ubuntu" in South Africa, is an underlying value in indigenous African worldviews. **Ntu therapy** (Gregory & Harper, 2001) is an African-centered approach developed in the U.S. "Ntu" is a Bantu concept that means essence and refers to the universal energy of all that is. It stresses harmony, balance, interconnectedness, and authenticity. The African-American holiday of Kwanzaa celebrates seven principles that are part of the African cultural heritage and offers an opportunity for African-centered healing (Messias *et al.*, 2020). The principles are:

1. *Umoja* (Unity)
2. *Kujichagulia* (Self-Determination)
3. *Ujima* (Collective Work and Responsibility)
4. *Ujamaa* (Cooperative economics)
5. *Nia* (Purpose)
6. *Kuumba* (Creativity)
7. *Imani* (Faith): To believe with all our hearts in our people, our parents, our teachers, our leaders, and the righteousness and victory of our struggle.

9.10 Religiously Integrated Cognitive Behavioral Therapy

Religiously Integrated Cognitive Behavioral Therapy (Pearce *et al.*, 2015), is a manualized treatment for depression that has been developed for the four major religions (Christianity, Judaism, Buddhism and Hinduism). Its seven major tools are:

1. Renewing of the mind (changing one's thinking)
2. Scripture memorization
3. Contemplative prayer
4. Challenging thoughts using one's religious resources
5. Religious practices (e.g., gratitude, altruism, forgiveness)

6.   Religious/spiritual resources
7.   Involvement in religious community

9.11 Psychoactive substances, spirituality, and mental health

St. Arnaud & Cormier (2017) note that the use of psychoactive substances can result in either a psychotic disorder or a spiritual disorder, or both, since ingesting substance such as LSD, psilocybin, mescaline, ayahuasca, and other hallucinogenic drugs can provoke both psychotic symptoms and spiritual emergencies. They stress the importance of an accurate diagnosis because, though antipsychotics can be helpful in cases of psychosis, they can actually worsen a spiritual emergency. There are many who advocate for the use of psychoactive substances for treating a range of disorders including anxiety, depression, anorexia, and even addiction. Pollan (2019), in his discussion of the use of psychedelics in psychotherapy, argues that the primary explanation for the beneficial effects of psychedelics on anxiety and depression has to do with the fact that they result in the diminishing or dissolution of the ego. In 2019, Johns Hopkins, a leading medical research institution, announced the opening of their Center for Psychedelic and Consciousness Research. The purpose of this center is to study the effectiveness of compounds like LSD and psilocybin for a range of mental health problems, including anorexia, addiction, and depression. The center was the first of its kind in the country, established with $17 million in commitments from wealthy private donors and a foundation. Cannabis, which is now legal in many jurisdictions, may have many of the same effects (Earlywine *et al.*, 2021). Reiff *et al.* (2020) have reviewed the evidence-based literature on psychedelic-assisted psycho-therapy and have concluded that the published scientific evidence, while limited, supports continued experimental research on the usefulness of psy-chedelic drugs for the treatment of mental illnesses but does not yet support the use of any of these drugs for patient care by mental health professionals outside of research settings. Cashwell *et al.* (2007) use Wellwood's term "spir-itual bypass" to refer to attempts to resolve psychological issues at the spirit-ual level exclusively, thus avoiding the necessary and challenging work of resolving them emotionally. The use of psychedelics can enable spiritual bypass by creating altered moods that enable the user to escape psychological pain.

Plante (2009, p. 33) offers "thirteen tools for your psychotherapeutic toolbox". These can be used across the range of client spiritual orientations and religious beliefs:

1. Prayer
2. Meditation
3. Meaning, purpose, and calling in life
4. Bibliotherapy (the reading of specific texts for the purpose of healing)
5. Attending community services and rituals
6. Volunteerism and charity
7. Ethical values and behavior
8. Forgiveness, gratitude, and kindness
9. Social justice
10. Learning from spiritual models
11. Acceptance of self and others (even with faults)
12. Being part of something larger than oneself
13. Appreciating the sacredness of life

9.12 Polyvagal theory

Dana (2018) describes a number of tools that help to activate the ventral vagal system to enhance a client's sense of safety and connection. According to Porges' polyvagal theory (2019), ventral vagal system activation supports the spiritual experience. Tools include:

- Savoring: remembering and enjoying a positive moment from the past.
- SIFTing: the four elements of body sensation, image, emotional feeling, and thought are combined and given a name so that they can be used for ventral vagal activation in the future. Elements can be real or imagined events.
- Developing curiosity regarding new or different experiences to increase a sense of connection and safety.
- Reframing fear responses as a continuum and encouraging movement toward the safety end of the continuum.

- Viewing the same experience from the perspective of each of the three different states (flight/flight, freeze, and connection).

This chapter has presented a number of models for and approaches to spiritually based psychotherapy. Some incorporate the beliefs and practices and others do not. It is important to remember that there are many variations within each of these perspectives as they are applied. Research is typically necessary to learn more about a client's belief system and in many cases, one must seek supervision and, perhaps, consultation with clergy, other spiritual leaders, and other professionals. This issue will be discussed in the next chapter.

Discussion questions

1. Lannert (1991) has presented the following case: A 20-year-old college junior (presumably a Christian) reluctantly agreed to see a psychiatrist for feelings of depression and hostility which he had been struggling to control through prayer and Bible reading. He explained that much of his reluctance to seek help came from a previous experience with a psychiatrist who told him that his difficulties stemmed largely from "his being too religious". (His memory of this simplistic formulation was partially confirmed by a note from the first psychiatrist, who indicated that his treatment plan had "focused on the reduction of religious preoccupation".)

    What approach would you take in working with this young man? Why?

2. Mrs. J., a 53-year-old widow, had been depressed for a few months after the death of her husband. Although the marriage seemed happy at times, there were many stormy periods during their relationship. There had been no visible signs of grief since his death. Since the funeral, she had been depressed and had lost interest in her surroundings. For no apparent reason, she blamed herself for minor events of the past. Sometimes she criticized herself for traits that characterized her husband more than herself. She had had a similar reaction after the death of her mother 23 years previously, when she and her mother had lived together. From the history, it could be inferred that the relation was characterized by hostile dependency. Six months after the mother's death, the patient married. She seemed intelligent and motivated for treatment and had considered psychotherapy in the past to gain a better understanding of herself (Peteet, 2014).

Pick two different spiritually based approaches and compare how they would handle this.

3. Griffith (2012) tells the story of a "Mr. Rogers" who was diagnosed with major depression with psychotic features based on his current depressive symptoms, history of depression, and family history of depression. He brooded and ruminated over the guilt he felt for falling short as a husband, father, and Christian. He felt he deserved punishment and God's wrath. He refused antidepressant medication, believing that he should deal with his difficulties through self-discipline and faith in God. In addition, he wanted to avoid the embarrassment he would experience if his friends learned that he was seeing a psychiatrist and taking medication. In his local community people were expected to deal with emotional problems with family and pastoral support.

How would you build rapport with Mr. Rogers? What countertransferential issues do you think you might encounter?

4. What kinds of client issues, beliefs and practices are likely to trigger countertransference reactions in you? What are some coping mechanisms you can use in these situations?

Exercise

Try one of the meditation exercises provided in this handout: https://positivepsychology.com/meditation-exercises-activities/. Write several paragraphs describing your experience. How comfortable would you be teaching the meditation practice to a client?

Resources

The Office of Religious and Spiritual Life at the University of La Verne, in California, has published a listing of general and faith-based apps that can be used to enhance spiritual well-being: https://laverne.edu/chaplain/apps-for-spiritual-wellbeing/

Meditation exercises: https://positivepsychology.com/meditation-exercises-activities/

Guided meditations: https://www.tarabrach.com/guided-meditations/

Chapter 10

Age and Stage-related Issues and Interventions

Vieten & Scammell (2015) note that individual and family spiritual orientations change over the life cycle, with almost half of U.S. adults changing their religious affiliation at least once during their lifetime, usually in young adulthood, with most of those changing away from their childhood affiliation. Still, they note that 47% of adults report they have not changed their religious faith since childhood (Pew Forum on Religion and Public Life, 2009). Some of the changes that they identify are:

1. **Switching:** changing to a different denomination within the same religion
2. **Apostasy:** dropping out of one's religion never to return
3. **Conversion:** shifting to a new faith or belief system
4. **Deconversion:** dropping out of a previously chosen group
5. **Intensification:** a revitalized commitment to a religion
6. **Cycling:** repeatedly shifting religious affiliations of involvement dropping out of a religion and returning later, or periodically falling out of faith

They observe that even when people do not change their affiliations, they may change in other ways, including changes in their spiritual beliefs, the extent to which they internalize certain values, the frequency with which they attend church or other spiritual events, and the types of spiritual coping they use. Using Rambo's (1993) seven-stage model of religious conversion, she describes the factors that may shape changes in spiritual beliefs, practices, or affiliations:

1. **Context:** The sum total of the spiritual influences that have shaped the individual up to the present
2. **Crisis:** An event that destabilizes a person's spiritual beliefs or identity such as trauma, a sudden and painful discovery, illness, or the loss of a loved one
3. **Quest:** A search for helpful alternative approaches whether as a part of their faith tradition or not
4. **Encounter:** An encounter with someone who follows a particular spiritual path and who may become a mentor of some kind
5. **Interaction:** Interaction with a new spiritual or religious community
6. **Commitment:** Full participation in the new faith community
7. **Consequences:** Full commitment to the new faith

Vieten & Scammell point out that though conversion to a new faith or denomination can occur at any age, it most often occurs when people are in their teens and early 20s. They suggest inquiring further about the client's experience and possibly recommending that the client considering or undergoing conversion read about others who have changed their beliefs or affiliations to normalize their experience. They also caution that one cannot assume that psychological growth and spiritual growth are the same thing:

> An important distinction to make here is that changes in spiritual or religious beliefs or practices over a person's lifetime may not be the same as psychological growth. For example, some people may find profound contentment and a sense of meaning and purpose in religious or spiritual development while still facing unresolved psychological symptoms, such as anxiety, depression, or addiction. Conversely, people may experience psychological development over time with relatively little spiritual or religious growth.

10.1 Infancy and early childhood

The psychological capacities in infancy that lay the foundation for later spiritual development are secure attachment and basic trust. These are fostered by parenting practices that are responsive to the infant's needs. Interventions around attachment issues in infancy typically focus on parental education and, if necessary, parental or family psychotherapy. Naimi *et al.* (2021) found that a spiritual intervention could reduce the anxiety and stress of parents of hospitalized newborns which presumably facilitated infant attachment. There are also attachment-based therapeutic approaches that address attachment and trust issues from infancy and early childhood in older children and adults. These typically rely on establishing a secure bond between the child and the therapist which can be used to explore and work through attachment issues and later be generalized beyond the therapeutic relationship. Brisch (2014), whose approach is informed by psychodynamic theory, presents six guidelines for working with children's attachment issues, asserting that the mental health professional should:

1. Function as a reliable physical base in their caring behavior so that a secure attachment can develop.
2. Facilitate and observe symbolic play that relates to the child's experienced relationship to the attachment figures.
3. Interpret attachment-related interactions with the child either verbally or through symbolic play interactions.
4. Foster emotional expression related to the attachment issues and link them to past attachment issues.
5. Provide security-promoting attachment experiences.
6. Dissolve the therapeutic bond carefully so that it will serve as a model for handling separations (p. 105).

Therapeutic or supportive holding is sometimes used to provide a "corrective emotional experience" for a child with an attachment disorder, but this technique has often been misused in parent education and treatment programs by coupling it with involuntary restraint and is no longer permitted in many programs and facilities (Howe & Fearnley, 1999).

The important thing to remember about spiritually relevant interventions in infancy is that they must address the caregiver relationship to provide a responsive, nurturing, and stable parenting situation for the infant.

10.2 Childhood

While children's spiritual development has received a degree of attention in research and theory, very little is known about integrating spirituality into the assessment or treatment of children. Boynton & Mellan (2021) call attention to the relative absence of literature and training on spiritually integrated psychotherapy for children. They consider this especially unfortunate since mental health professionals are often called on to support children who have experienced trauma, grief or loss. They argue that access to the spiritual dimension can be a critical part of healing for these issues. In his classic study, Coles (1990) interviewed hundreds of children from Jewish, Christian, Muslim, Hopi, and secular homes and concluded that, like adults, all children look for answers to questions like "Where do we come from" and "What is the meaning of life", though they may not use these words. The way they think and talk about such questions is influenced by their age, vocabulary, and level of cognitive development.

Andrews & Marotta (2005) point out that the level of children's development influences how they conceptualize and cope with death and decry the failure of the literature to shed light on how developmental level affects the process or on the specific role of spirituality as a coping mechanism for grieving children. Coholic (2010) has authored a book for children coping with trauma, grief, or loss that includes art activities aimed at promoting mindfulness and spiritual awareness that is appropriate for use by mental health professionals who are not trained in art therapy. She points out that her activities not only aid in healing but also facilitate spiritually sensitive conversations between children and their therapist. She reports the following conversation between an art activities facilitator (Barb) and a child (Mary) who talked about the religious beliefs of her family and a Christian youth group she was attending (p. 73):

Mary: I don't know what's wrong with me. My heart is saying that I am Christian but my whole body is saying, no, you're not a Christian.

Barb: So you are really struggling then, finding out who you are?

Mary: Yeah.

Barb: How do you find what guides you or lets you feel like your true self?

Mary: I don't know what guides me. I don't know.

Barb: How do you think you are going to figure that out?

Mary: Maybe I will understand when I am older.

Barb: Yes, and maybe through some of the activities where we talk about ourselves. Maybe that will help you learn more about yourself too.

Pandya (2018b) has reported the results of a large-scale, two-year-long, cross-cultural, controlled study of a spiritually focused intervention for children diagnosed with anxiety disorders. Four themes were covered in the intervention:

1. Connecting with the God within
2. Recognizing and annihilating fear through introspection and breathing
3. Stilling and centering
4. Cultivating a balanced and calm consciousness

The study found that the intervention reduced anxiety, especially in girls, children from the more affluent cities, and those who attended more sessions than required and practiced at home.

10.3 Adolescence

Adolescence is marked by the emergence of abstract reasoning and, ideally, is a time for forming a stable and positive sense of identity. Magaldi-Dopman & Park-Taylor (2013) highlight six concerns that are often relevant for adolescents:

1. The relationship between spirituality/religion and health and coping
2. Negotiating multiple social identities
3. Religious cults
4. Religious conversion experiences
5. Anti-religious sentiment or religious discrimination
6. Ethical considerations

They urge psychotherapists to reassure adolescents that it is safe to talk about these issues in therapy. Mindfulness training has been shown to be useful in helping adolescents deal with stress and anxiety around identity and other issues (Lucas-Thompson *et al.*, 2019). An experimental study has shown that Spiritual Components Training, an Islamic-based program, enhanced the life satisfaction of Persian adolescents (Rouholamini *et al.*, 2017). Adolescents often question or abandon their family's religious traditions. This can result in family conflict. Çetintaş & Ekşi (2020) point out that spiritual-oriented family therapy can be helpful in resolving these issues.

Spiritual interventions can be useful in treating specific issues in adolescents. Rickhi *et al.* (2015) evaluated an eight-week online spirituality informed e-mental health intervention for adolescent **depression** that guided participants through an exploration of spiritually informed principles such as forgiveness, gratitude, and compassion. They found the intervention to be effective in reducing mild to moderate major depression. This improvement was retained at follow-up. Jackson *et al.* (2010) examined spirituality, beliefs about spirituality, and participation in spiritual activities in 180 foster care youth from diverse racial and ethnic backgrounds. They found that over 95% of them believed in God and 79% considered prayer a spiritual practice. Most said that love and forgiveness have helped them heal. Based on the value these youth ascribed to spiritual coping mechanisms, the authors recommended that spirituality be integrated into practice and caregiving for youth in foster care. Adelson *et al.* (2019) point to the mental health stressors faced by lesbian, gay, bisexual, and transgender (**LGBT**) youth. They are at risk for suicide, bias-related victimization, stress, family rejection, and stigma and must struggle with self-acceptance and decisions about whether to "come out". They argue that health care chaplains are in a unique position to help LGBT youth and their families to address issues of whether or not their spiritual/religious tradition is affirming or non-accepting of the young person's orientation or gender identity. By demonstrating respect for the family's religious beliefs while supporting the youth's well-being, they can contribute to the assessment of salient religious/spiritual factors, collaborate with child psychiatrists to support coping with mental health risk factors, including anti-LGBT stigma, discourage "conversion therapy", and recognize the youth's gender identity and preference.

Spiritual tools can also help both children and adolescents cope with **trauma**. The concept of "**posttraumatic growth**" has become popular in the last several decades. The term was coined by psychologists Tedeschi & Calhoun (2004) to refer to positive psychological growth that can occur in the process of struggling with a traumatic event. They also developed an inventory to measure posttraumatic growth. The factors they report were: improved relationships to others, a sense of new possibilities, increased personal strength, spiritual change, and greater appreciation of life. Prieto-Ursúa & Jódar (2020) observe that making sense of or finding meaning in traumatic events can promote spiritual growth and that spiritual or religious beliefs and values can help in the search for meaning. In their study of reactions to the coronavirus they found that both spirituality and religiosity were positively related to posttraumatic growth. Taku & McDiarmid (2015) have confirmed the capacity for posttraumatic growth in adolescents and its positive effects on self-esteem. Tedeschi (2020) suggests the following interventions to facilitate posttraumatic growth:

1. Educate the client regarding psychological effects of trauma
2. Suggest techniques to regulate emotions such as observation, exercise, and meditation
3. Support the client as they tell the story
4. Suggest the client engage in service helping others who have experienced similar traumas

O'Neill (2020) has reviewed the literature on expressive arts therapy and found that such therapy is especially powerful in reducing symptoms of trauma in adolescent girls.

Adolescence is an important time for questioning and self-definition and, regardless of the issues they present in therapy, it is important to provide a welcoming reception to their spiritual concerns and coping resources.

10.4 Adulthood

Challenges in adulthood include establishing independence, forming viable relationships and work roles, and nurturing offspring or in other ways beginning to leave a legacy for the future (generativity). Questioning of one's spiritual beliefs may also occur in adulthood, especially when spiritual growth makes earlier beliefs seem too rigid or limiting. Nelson (2009) points out that a common event in young adulthood or midlife is a **turning point**:

> Something that redirects our life on a long-lasting basis. This could include changes or recommitments in roles or important goals as family members die, or we experience failures in relationships and careers… Midlife turning points can be sudden affairs provoked by a crisis or struggle, but more commonly they involve a slow steady acceptance of changes that lead toward increasing responsibility and maturity… Turning points are often only recognized in retrospect and can be experienced initially as a feeling of estrangement or as a sense of acedia — discontent, apathy or boredom — rather than severe emotional turmoil, depression, or anxiety (p. 280).

He notes the strong link between spirituality and generativity and emphasizes the value of spiritually based interventions for supporting those who have reached a turning point. He also advocates the use of narrative techniques helping individuals craft life stories that make sense of the changes they have undergone. Such stories can include the following kinds of events:

- Originating events that provide a cornerstone for ideology and belief
- Anchoring events that direct the person and provide life lessons
- Transitional events that cannot be understood within the context of the story
- Crisis or limit events that force a reappraisal and new understanding through inner and social dialogue

Spiritual involvement is also helpful in promoting posttraumatic growth in adults who have experienced trauma, either in their adult lives or earlier (Reinert *et al.*, 2016).

10.5 Older adulthood

The World Values Survey Association (2014) has collected data on major countries with different religious traditions and degrees of secularization. In almost all countries, those 60 and over are more likely to report that they are religious. Though there is little research on spirituality and psychological well-being in older adults, Zimmer *et al.* (2016), based on a literature review, report that there is a positive relationship between religiosity and mental health in older adults and that prayer and meditation have been found useful in relieving stress and promoting well-being in this population. They note that, as in other age groups, religion can have negative effects on mental health when it fosters negative attitudes such as guilt or shame, when it demands unquestioning devotion and obedience, when it substitutes faith healing for medical care, or when interactions with other members of the faith community are unfavorable. Spiritual organizations and practices can be valuable in reducing social isolation, encouraging healthy behavior, providing mechanisms for coping with stress, and promoting healthy exercises such as forgiveness. A study carried out by Stanley *et al.* (2011) found that most older adults prefer including religion and/or spirituality in psychotherapy for anxiety and depression. The study participants were mostly Christian and most indicated that religion or spirituality played an important role in their lives at present. Those who already used positive religious-based coping were the most likely to prefer religiously/spiritually based interventions in therapy. Based on these findings, Barrera *et al.* (2012) developed a cognitive behavioral manualized treatment protocol called "Calmer Life" that could be administered with or without spiritually based elements. For example, in the spiritually inclusive protocol, clients engaging in the deep breathing and progressive muscle relaxation modules may be asked to focus on a religious image or word while they practice the exercises. Both life review and Jungian shadow work (see Chapter 5) can be useful processes for older adults.

For those elderly individuals who are experiencing increased disability and frailty, gerotranscendence becomes an issue. How do they find meaning, value, and hope in life in spite of their diminishing faculties? Çetintaş & Ekşi (2020) note that family therapists can provide family caregivers with the opportunity to make sense of positive and negative spiritual experiences that affect the well-being of those for whom they care and can provide new resources for care if care demands increase. Mowat (2011) reports on the positive effects of spiritual care for people with dementia, pointing out the importance of relationship-building, storytelling, listening, and creating space for conversations to take place. McKinlay (2006) has listed 14 spiritual needs of physically ill elders based on an earlier work by Koenig *et al.* (2004):

1. The need for meaning, purpose, and hope
2. The need to transcend circumstances
3. The need for support in dealing with loss
4. The need for continuity
5. The need for validation and support of religious behaviors
6. The need to engage in religious behaviors
7. The need for personal dignity and a sense of worthiness
8. The need for unconditional love
9. The need to express anger and doubt
10. The need to feel that God is on their side
11. The need to love and serve others
12. The need to be thankful
13. The need to forgive and be forgiven
14. The need to prepare for death and dying

Hodge *et al.* (2010) caution that a distinction must be made between psychotherapy and spiritual direction when working with older adults, cautioning that mental health professionals can inadvertently fall into the role of spiritual director when exploring spirituality with their clients but that this role is outside their area of competence. Where spiritual growth is the primary focus, clients should be referred to pastoral counselors or clergy.

10.6 Death and dying

Coyle (2004) has coined the term "existential slap" to refer to the experience of truly comprehending, on a gut level, that death is imminent. The process of dying, in addition to physical pain, often also evokes psychological, social, and spiritual suffering (Callahan, 2017). She points out that in a study of dying patients, Yang *et al.* (2010) found that while most of the patients were able to adapt to their new reality, this adaptation required the patients to manage intense emotions connected to living within a meaningless void before they could come to accept that death was inevitable. Callahan uses Pesut's (2008) classification of spiritual care into monistic, theistic, and humanistic to discuss how dying patients may be able to find meaning in their experience. A monistic perspective assumes that all things and people are connected. The prospect of death may cause the individual to feel as if they are part of something larger than themselves. For clients who feel this way, activities such as meditation or being outdoors can be helpful. A theistic perspective focuses on a transcendent relationship to a divine higher power. If these are the client's religious beliefs then religious rites of worship may be important and it is important to involve a formal spiritual care provider. A humanistic perspective emphasizes the need for the individual to experience an awareness of life's meaning and purpose.

Though there are age differences in the kinds of life challenges that individuals confront and the spiritual resources they have available to cope with these challenges, we are all, as Harry Stack Sullivan is so often quoted as saying, "much more simply human than otherwise". Compassion, caring, and empathy are always appropriate and human connection can be one of the most important resources for humans, regardless of their age or condition. The next chapter will discuss how working with other professionals and community practitioners can enhance a mental health professional's spiritual competence.

Discussion questions

For each of the case vignettes below describe the questions you would ask to determine the client's perspective and resources. What age- or stage-related issues do you think might be involved in each of the cases?

1. Renee is a 41-year-old married woman from a town that experienced heavy damage from a tornado that killed her 16-year-old son when his school collapsed. Renee is now seven months pregnant with her second child and has sought psychotherapy because she does not feel she will be able to overcome her grief and she is obsessed with fears for her new baby.

2. Arnold is a 66-year-old retired gay man who has been HIV-positive since he was a young man. He is single and lives alone. He was recently diagnosed with stage-4 liver cancer and, at the urging of his parents, who are still alive, has agreed to see a therapist because he does not want to undertake chemotherapy treatment for his cancer.

3. Peter is a 19-year-old male college student who is suffering from Traumatic Brain Injury following a motor vehicle accident six months ago in which he was a passenger. He has been having trouble regulating his behavior and managing his college studies since the accident and has been lethargic and irritable at home. Though his parents are warm and supportive, he has had periodic outbursts of anger toward them. He has been resistant to his therapist regarding how to improve his attention span and impulse control.

Exercise

Use the internet to research evidence-based parenting interventions and training programs that promote parent-child attachment. Write a few paragraphs on what you have found.

Resource

Stages and issues over the family life cycle: https://wps.ablongman.com/wps/media/objects/4915/5033208/Fourth_ed.pdf

Chapter 11

Professional Considerations

Spiritual competence for mental health professionals includes being able to collaborate effectively with professionals from other disciplines, especially other health, allied health, and behavioral health care professionals, clergy, and other pastoral workers. There are also circumstances in which it can be helpful for mental health professionals to refer to or collaborate with healers or spiritual leaders outside the professional structure of the Western medical system or local licensing structure. This chapter presents a model for such collaboration and reviews existing training programs focusing on interprofessional collaboration in spiritual care.

Consultation involves interaction between a mental health professional and another professional, practitioner, or spiritual leader. It is common to distinguish between client-centered consultation and consultee-centered consultation (Caplan *et al.*, 1995). **Client-centered consultation** involves seeking the opinion of another practitioner regarding a client's progress, issues and/or treatment. **Consultee-centered consultation** focuses on the personal and/or professional issues of an individual practitioner, or the administration and staffing of the practice site, insofar as they may be interfering with clinical or ethical integrity. Consultation may be sought either by or from the mental health professional. **Collaboration** is an ongoing form of periodic consultation focused on the client's mental health and/or spiritual issues. Bilich *et al.* (2000) distinguish between limited and full collaboration. In **limited collaboration**, the mental health professional sees the client for psychotherapy while the collaborating professional or practitioner sees the client for their specialty and the two maintain regular contact. In **full collaboration**, the collaborators plan their work together and meet regularly with one another. They may meet regularly or periodically together with the client. The therapist may also consider referral to a pastoral counselor or other faith-based mental health professionals. **Referral** occurs when a mental health professional recommends that a client seek another provider or when another provider recommends that a client with whom they are working see a mental health professional.

Outreach and education in spiritual communities can also be important in educating clergy and faith-based organizations regarding mental illness and its treatment and overcoming cultural barriers to seeking help from a mental health professional. In their discussion of collaboration between Black churches and mental health professions, Dempsey *et al.* (2016) give several reasons why African Americans may seek mental health support from their church rather than the mental health system:

- It is free of charge.
- They are already familiar with and may have a relationship with the pastoral worker.
- They are more comfortable engaging with someone of their own race and culture.
- The church experience itself provides therapeutic release and restores faith and hope.

They list eight "best practices" for mental health professionals when reaching out to clergy and congregations:

1. Cultural awareness and competence
2. Understanding church etiquette and hierarchy
3. Approval from the church leader
4. Participation in church health fairs
5. Provision of mental health training for church leadership
6. Becoming an active member of the church community
7. Conduct needs assessment research
8. Include church leaders on advisory boards of mental health organizations

Barnett & Johnson (2011) present the following case as an example of the importance of seeking clinical supervision, considering referral, and/or consulting or collaborating with other professionals or practitioners (with the client's appropriate consent) when a clinician is faced with a clinical or ethical dilemma, when it would be in the client's best interest, or when requested by the client:

> A 35-year-old stay-at-home mother is a victim of persistent domestic violence. She is an intelligent and insightful psychotherapy client but resists any discussion of leaving her spouse, or even becoming more assertive, on the basis of her "biblical duty" to remain obedient to her husband. She quotes passages of scripture that emphasize a wife's obligation to remain under her husband's authority. The psychotherapist feels quite uncomfortable about the client's religious rationale for remaining in what is seen as an abusive and unhealthy relationship. She wonders about involving the client's priest in psychotherapy to leverage change but is unsure about how to proceed (p. 155).

A first step in this case would be to seek clinical supervision. The possibility of the client, the therapist, or both consulting with the client's priest should be discussed in supervision and perhaps next with the client. If consultation with the priest does not help the therapist and the client agree on a treatment plan, the therapist should discuss referral with her clinical supervisor.

11.1 Clinical supervision

It is unfortunate that the literature on clinical supervision for mental health professionals who are working with their clients on spiritually related issues is scant, since supervision is a primary resource in these situations. Even less has been written about the use of spiritual disciplines in supervision. Supervision regarding spiritual issues in therapy is called for by all professional ethical codes with provisions for cultural and/or spiritual competence and occurs along the same lines as general clinical supervision. Shafranske (2014) presents a number of suggestions and guidelines for the clinical supervision of mental health professionals in the area of spirituality. Shafranske recommends that what he calls R/S (religion and spirituality) competence be explicitly included in the supervision contract and that the supervisory discussion be informed by the four following conclusions from the research literature:

1. Religious coping is often turned to in extreme circumstances when other resources have been exhausted.
2. Religious coping is most effective when R/S is internalized, intrinsically motived, and situated within a congruent community.
3. There are advantages and disadvantages to even the most controversial forms of religion.
4. Use of R/S resources does not always have a positive effect on mental health.

He recommends that supervisors contribute to supervising skill development by:

1. Promoting introspection, self-assessment, and awareness of how personal beliefs, values, and worldview affect interaction with clients.
2. Self-assessment of their own relevant knowledge, skills, and values.
3. Reviewing, applying, and discussing with the supervisee the ethical principles associated with spiritually integrative treatment.
4. Closely monitoring any interventions addressing R/S and explore supervisee and client reactions, ensuring that client preferences were elicited and informed consent was obtained to address R/S in treatment.
5. Modeling respect for the supervisee's autonomy by limiting inquiry to R/S attitudes and values that directly affect the supervisee's therapeutic interactions with the client.

Ross *et al.* (2013) have synthesized a unified model of how spirituality can be addressed in supervision based on a literature review. They call this model SACRED for: **S**afety (informed consent), **A**ssessment, **C**onceptualization (learning about other spiritual worldviews, incorporating religious and spiritual themes, recognizing and overcoming countertransference), **R**eflection (on how to apply knowledge clinically and personally), **E**merging congruence (promoting congruence between the religious or spiritual issues and the presenting issues), and **D**evelopment (continued learning and development). Miller *et al.* (2007) have developed a "Spiritual Issues in Supervision Scale" in which various issue areas are rated on a 5-point Likert scale according to how often they are addressed in supervision.

11.2 Referral

The provider to or from whom the client is referred may be another mental health professional, a member of the clergy, or another indigenous, complementary, or alternative provider. The referral may involve either the continuation or the termination of the relationship between the client and the source of the referral. The *Preliminary Practice Guidelines for Working with Religious and Spiritual Issues* from the American Psychological Association's Division of Spirituality and Religion (Hathaway & Ripley, 2009) state that the need for clinical referral based on religious/spiritual factors is suggested when:

- The client expresses a strong preference for a therapist with a different religious/spiritual background and this preference persists after reasonable attempts are made to establish rapport with the client.
- The presenting problem requires an understanding of the client's religious/spiritual background that exceeds the psychologist's competence regardless of relevant consultation or supervision.
- A religious/spiritual difference between the client and the psychologist impedes treatment (p. 49).

Ethical practice requires that a mental health professional who terminates a relationship with a client must provide an appropriate referral (this is not necessary if the client initiates the termination although referrals may still be made). Referrals do not require interaction between the provider to whom the client is referred and the therapist, though it is often helpful to make contact to assess provider fit and availability.

11.3 Working with clergy and other spiritual leaders

Koenig *et al.* (2020) give an example of a successful collaboration between a Muslim imam and a psychiatrist:

> The client, Bakir, is a 58-year-old lawyer who is a member of his mosque and suffers from severe anxiety because he is afraid that his "bad deeds" outweigh his "good deeds" and he will spend eternity in hell. The imam has suggested spiritual practices and given practical advice but Bakir's anxiety has only worsened. The imam suggested that Bakir see a psychiatrist and,

with Bakir's permission, speaks to the psychiatrist before the appointment to explain the situation to him. The psychiatrist gives Bakir prescriptions for medications, but Bakir is worried that the medication may be contrary to his religious belief that he should rely on God alone. The psychiatrist refers him back to the imam, who reassures him that it is okay to take the medication. Bakir's anxiety improves.

Cooperation between mental health professionals on the one hand, and clergy and other spiritual leaders on the other, has been recommended from both clinical and clerical perspectives, but mutual mistrust, stigma, and time constraints can present barriers. Studies in several countries indicate that though clergy and other spiritual leaders may consider themselves important in assisting members of their community with mental health issues, they are unlikely to avail themselves of the opportunity to refer, consult, or collaborate with mental health professionals (e.g., Freire *et al.*, 2019; Helestine-Carp & Hoskins, 2020). Barriers to cooperation may be more powerful in some professional situations and religious and spiritual communities than others. Dempsey *et al.* (2016), for example, point out that African Americans are more likely to seek support from their church than from mental health professionals. The American Psychiatric Association (2018) has published a mental health guide for faith leaders that can be a valuable resource for clinicians to share with clergy when they are working together. It includes the following explanation:

> A person might express to either a clinician or more likely to a faith leader experiences such as receiving a message from "God", punishment for sin, a calling to a "great holy cause", possession by "evil spirits", or persecution because of a conviction of "spiritual closeness". It is important to distinguish whether these are symptoms of a mental disorder (for example, delusions, auditory or visual hallucinations, and paranoia), distressing experiences of a religious or spiritual problem, or both. Mental health illnesses that may have symptoms with a religious or spiritual content include psychotic disorders (for example, schizophrenia, schizoaffective disorder), mood disorders (for example, major depression, bipolar disorders), and substance use disorders, among others. Also, for a person of faith, having a mental illness may be seen as a spiritual concern or problem, just as having cancer or a heart attack would (p. 7).

Collaboration between mental health professionals and clergy or spiritual leaders can be especially important when the client is struggling with an issue that is stigmatized by their spiritual community. Adelson *et al.* (2019), for example, point out the value of such collaboration for LGBT youth.

11.4 Working with other providers

There are mental health professionals who are trained in both psychotherapy and spiritual or pastoral counseling. Pastoral counselors are clergy members with training in clinical pastoral education. They are trained to diagnose and provide counseling. Pastoral counselors can have equivalents to a doctorate in counseling. There are also psychotherapists who have been trained in spiritually integrated psychotherapy or in a specific faith-based therapeutic approach. Using a biopsychospiritual model can involve working with an interdisciplinary team that includes only mental health professionals and clergy or other spiritual leaders or healers. Schultz *et al.* (2014) stress the importance of the following for interdisciplinary team effectiveness:

- Shared goals and values
- Shared team culture
- Open communication
- Understanding and respect for the competencies of other team members
- Equal value and regard for each member's contributions
- Willingness to learn from those with different perspectives
- Clarity on individual professional and legal accountability

Researchers interviewing mental health workers and clergy after a mine disaster in West Virginia (Curtis *et al.*, 2017), to learn more about how they collaborated and what facilitated their collaboration, found four factors that contributed to effective collaboration:

1. Mutual respect
2. Pre-established relationships
3. Mental health professionals' sensitivity to religious/spiritual issues
4. Clergy members' training in disaster spiritual and emotional care

11.5 Expressive therapies

Expressive therapies can be helpful for clients who are struggling with spiritual issues. Land (2015) suggests that this may be because expressive methods access the spiritual realm more easily than verbal and abstract reasoning. Expressive therapies include, but are not limited to, the following specialty areas: art, writing, music, drama and psychodrama, dance and movement, poetry or bibliotherapy, and play therapy. The minimum training to be an expressive therapist is a master's degree plus some training in the art form itself. There are several professional associations that certify expressive therapists, some international. Expressive therapies facilitate psychological healing at a non-verbal level and some expressive therapy approaches incorporate spirituality (e.g., Horovitz, 2017). Expressive therapies can be recommended as adjunctive treatments with or without therapist collaboration.

11.6 Complementary and alternative medicine

The U.S. National Institutes of Health (2021) defines complementary and alternative medicine as follows: "Medical products and practices that are not part of standard medical care". Standard medical care varies among cultures but can be defined as "treatment that is accepted by medical experts as a proper treatment for a certain type of disease and that is widely used by healthcare professionals" (*ibid*). Complementary medicine is used alongside standard medical care while alternative medicine is used in place of such medicine. The National Institutes of Health has a special institute, the Institute for Complementary and Alternative Medicine, that studies five categories of such treatments:

1. Mind-body therapies that combine mental focus, breathing and body movements such as meditation, yoga, imagery, or expressive arts
2. Biologically based practices such as vitamins, supplements, botanical, or special diets
3. Manipulative and body-based practices such as massage, chiropractic therapy, or reflexology
4. Biofield therapy, sometimes called energy medicine, such as Reiki, acupuncture, or therapeutic touch
5. Whole medical systems such as Ayurvedic medicine, traditional Chinese medicine, homeopathy, or naturopathy

Because many forms of complementary and alternative medicine are not subject to the same kinds of regulatory standards as standard medical practitioners, practices, or medicines, it is important to invite clients' trust in confiding their own use of non-standard methods and to inform oneself regarding the safety of the techniques they use.

Complementary and alternative medicine play a crucial role in many societies today. Qureshi *et al.* (2018), for example, document their widespread use in Saudi Arabia. Lüddeckens (2018) argues that these approaches attract many because they do not distinguish between the biomedical and the spiritual and provide both kinds of care. Furthermore, they are less institutionalized, permitting the provider to be more responsive to client needs, and it is therefore more empowering to the client.

Hoskins & Platt (2021) point out that collaboration between mental health professionals and indigenous healers is rare and impeded by substantial mistrust. Few mental health training programs provide information on how clinicians might integrate concepts related to indigenous healing practices into their methods or collaborate with traditional healers. Yasir Abbasi, a South Asian Muslim psychiatrist in England, tells the following story (2016):

> "I am already dead! I have been buried,' said a young South Asian girl on the psychiatric ward. Prior to her admission she had stopped going to school, and instead isolated herself in her room spending hours on the internet searching for her grave. She was not eating much and losing weight. There had been occasions when she wandered off at night. With poor eye contact and slow speech, she added: "I can feel the worms crawling inside my body."

After an assessment she was found to have developed a severe form of depression with Cotard syndrome (a rare mental illness in which the affected person holds the delusional belief that he or she is already dead). Her family thought that the girl was possessed by a jinn and wanted to take her out of the hospital and bring her to a spiritual healer. Abassi met with the spiritual healer so that the healer could explain to the family the nature of the mental health problems. The family agreed to allow her to continue treatment in the hospital and they placed spiritual amulets around the room. The girl recovered and was discharged.

Kpobi & Swartz (2019) have studied the beliefs and practices of Muslim traditional healers in Ghana. These healers attribute mental illness and health to the workings of evil spirits, or jinn, and treat the mentally ill with a combination of Islamic and indigenous practices. People in Ghana often prefer to go to traditional healers because of their beliefs, and the fact that these providers are accessible and affordable. They found a deep commitment on the part of the traditional healers to non-maleficence, or the concept of "do no harm".

De Rios (2002), a medical anthropologist and licensed counselor, has argued that there is much that mental health professionals can learn from indigenous healers. She studied several indigenous healing techniques in Peru and has used them in Peru and with Latino clients in the U.S. The first difference she notes between psychotherapy and indigenous healing is that indigenous interventions are relatively brief, while psychotherapy typically occurs over a more extended period. Briefer interventions can reduce dropout rates among Latino immigrant populations. Second, indigenous healers often establish a highly suggestible trance state with their client enabling their suggestions to be more readily followed. Hypnosis can also be an option in psychotherapy. She noticed that the indigenous healers she observed were inclined to boast about their credentials and their successful cure rates. She suggests that mental health professionals who do not already do this frame their diplomas, licenses, and award certificates, and hang them on the walls of their office. She also urges them to mention, safeguarding their confidentiality, of course, of clients they have successfully treated.

In a South African study of psychiatrists' views of spiritual collaboration, Van Rensburg *et al.* (2014) allude to the fact that:

> …most of the international medical literature reflects North American and European authors' views, in which the discussion of the role of a religious or spiritual adviser in multidisciplinary health teams refers mostly to a Christian pastoral counsellor with additional experience or qualifications in clinical settings.

In an effort to eliminate limitations on religion imposed by colonial powers, the South African constitution affirms that no single faith tradition can be considered to have preference over others. As a result, South African mental health care teams lack formal guidelines on what training and experience in clinical conditions are needed for religious or spiritual advisors to qualify for such collaboration.

11.7 Working in faith-based organizations

Crisp (2014) defines a faith-based organization as one that derives its mission and identity from the teachings of one or more religious or spiritual traditions and/or "is under the auspices of a religious organization or community". Such setting may be especially appealing to mental health professionals who share their faith tradition but can be challenging for those who do not. She also points out that being of the same faith in a faith-based organization assures compatibility of beliefs and values, quoting a social worker in Jewish social service agency who said: "There are many shades of grey in being Jewish … there are secular Jews right through to sort of Orthodox Jews." While staff in a faith-based organization may not be required to share its religion, there still may be expectations about shared values. Crisp lists some areas in which ethical dilemmas may occur for the mental health professional:

- Sexual behavior and reproduction
- Medical interventions including blood transfusions, use of donor organs, and euthanasia
- Substance abuse, including alcohol or caffeine
- Beliefs about spirit possession, circumcision, corporal punishment, children's rights, and women's rights

Also, because of particular beliefs, faith-based organizations may choose not to provide certain services or to provide them within limited parameters. Crisp points out that ethical considerations may vary among religions. Citing Linzer (2006), Crisp says:

> For example, if an elderly person in care decided she no longer wanted to live and refused food, respect for autonomous choices may guide practitioners working in Protestant or Hindu settings, whereas the principle of sanctity of life would present issues in Catholic, Jewish and Muslim settings, all of which are religions which may consider such actions to be suicide, which is morally reprehensible.

Because most ethical guidelines for mental health professions call both for responsibility to the employer and respect for the autonomy of the client, clinicians in such settings can face ethical dilemmas and should seek supervision when they occur. Xu (2020) provides an interesting account of constraints in faith-based service organizations in China. While such organizations are now permitted, the government requires that professional workers be aligned with the Communist Party and assist the Party and the government to resolve social conflicts. This can create dilemmas for mental health professionals in these settings.

Discussion questions

How would you approach the spiritual issues raised in each of the following three cases? Describe what kinds of supervision or consultation you would seek, if any, and why (or why not). Would you make a referral? Would you need to do any research? If so, what would you need to learn about?

1. Vieten & Scammell (2015) tell the following story about a psychotherapist (Shelley) and her client (Barbara): Barbara had converted to a very conservative Christian sect before they first began working together. The therapy focused on work-related issues, not religious ones, but as they worked together for over a year, Barbara repeatedly mentioned going to church and attending special Bible-study classes. Shelly had a statue of Quan Yin (a Chinese goddess) in her office. To her it represented a feminine aspect of the sacred. One day Barbara came in furious, saying the statue deeply disturbed her and she wanted it removed. Shelley removed the statue immediately and listened to Barbara rage, learning that Barbara had been angry about this for a long time and nearly left her as a therapist because of it (pp. 24–25).

2. Ayesha is a Muslim adolescent who takes her religion very seriously, but because she has struggled with an eating disorder, for which she is currently seeing a psychotherapist, her doctor has told her that she should not fast during Ramadan, the month in which Muslims do not eat between sunrise and sunset. The doctor told her that research indicates that fasting can aggravate an eating disorder or, if it is remission, trigger a relapse. Ayesha tells her therapist that she plans to fast anyway because it is her religious duty.

3. John is a 45-year-old accountant who suffers from a severe anxiety disor-
    der. He has heard and read that cannabis-assisted therapy can be effective
    in treating anxiety disorders. It can be purchased and used legally in his
    state without a prescription and he tells his psychotherapist that he is
    planning to obtain and use marijuana to help with his anxiety. He would
    like to discuss his experiences with marijuana in therapy and obtain
    feedback from his therapist.

Exercise

Building a network of relationships with spiritually competent providers for
supervision, consultation, or referral will increase your resource base and
enhance your competence. Begin a file of such providers with whom you are
already familiar, indicating, for each provider:

1. Their area(s) of expertise and training
2. Certification and/or licensure
3. Their contact information
4. Your comments and a log of your contacts with them

If you do not already have any such relationships, contact three different
providers in any of the areas listed in the preceding chapter and use them to
begin your list.

Resources

National Institutes of Health, Center for Complementary and Integrative Health:
https://www.nccih.nih.gov/

The Mental Health and Faith Community Partnership: https://www.
psychiatry.org/psychiatrists/cultural-competency/engagement-opportunities/
mental-health-and-faith-community-partnership

Certification vs. Accreditation vs. Licensure: What's the Difference in Health Care?:
https://www.aeseducation.com/blog/certification-accreditation-licensure-
whats-the-difference-in-health-care

Chapter 12

Where Do We Go from Here?

This concluding chapter suggests some directions for the further development and improvement of spiritual competence in mental health care: decolonizing mental health perspectives, promoting holistic views of mental health, advancing the evidence-based research base, integrating spirituality into mental health practice and training, and working with clergy and faith-based communities.

12.1 Decolonizing mental health and mental health care

Watters (2010) gives numerous examples of the cultural insensitivity of Western aid workers' attempts to prevent and treat posttraumatic stress disorder in Sri Lanka in the wake of the 2004 tsunami. In the Western perspective, trauma is viewed as producing internal psychological damage which is treated by processing, or "working through", the experience. In Sri Lanka, the damage was seen as the loss of social connections. Western interventions focused on the individual rather than helping people and families reconnect and help each other. Moreover, symptoms of stress in individuals were not presented as psychological complaints but rather as somatic symptoms, resulting in multiple diagnostic errors. In another example drawn from research on indigenous and Western treatments for schizophrenia in Zanzibar, he describes how the biomedical model of schizophrenia can actually interfere with healing for people with schizophrenia in collectivist cultures that emphasize group over individual well-being. He cites World Health Organization studies showing that individuals diagnosed with schizophrenia in developing countries fare better than those in the industrialized world. The traditional view of what is called schizophrenia in the Western world is that it results from spirit possession and is not perceived as something abnormal or pathological. In contrast to mental illness, spirit possession is not stigmatized. Family members who see it as spirit possession are more accepting and non-judgmental in their attitudes toward the affective individual and do not pressure them to behave more "normally". He cites Mcgruder's (1999) anthropological studies in Zanzibar showing that individuals with schizophrenia whose families viewed schizophrenia as resulting from spirit possession were less likely to relapse.

Manjapra (2020) asserts: "The work of freeing consciousness from the ongoing effects of colonialism is still unfinished work." She points to the global and ongoing assembly of divergent post-colonial groups such as the 2018 gathering in Senegal where groups from 25 African countries came together to ask for an end to the "one-way humanitarianism" of Western NGOs. Lewis *et al.* (2018) advocate decolonizing mental health services in order to provide spiritually appropriate mental health care to care to indigenous people. In her paper, she applies the term as is customary, to the original inhabitants of a geographic area, in this case, to Native Americans in the U.S. Chakkarath (2013) and other "postcolonialists" use the term more broadly to refer native inhabitants of a region that has historically been colonized by Western powers, including his country of India. Gone (2008) has called the colonial imposition of Western mental health practices and concepts a form of "cultural proselytization" that persists in the neocolonialism of today. Mental health care providers and researchers in other countries have also spoken out in favor of incorporating indigenous approaches into mental health care. In 1982, Yang & Wen wrote:

> The subjects whom we studied are Chinese people in Chinese society, but, the theories and methods we used are mostly imported from the West or of the Western style. In our daily life, we are Chinese; when we are doing research, we become Western people. We repress our Chinese thoughts or philosophy intentionally or unintentionally and make them unable to be expressed in our procedure of research. … Under such a situation, we can only follow the West step by step with an expectation to catch up their academic trend. … Eventually, our existence in the world community of social and behavioral science becomes invisible at all (p. ii).

In a later work, Yang (1997) gives three reasons for promoting indigenous approaches in mental health care (pp. 236–262):

1. Specific findings of psychological research often do not replicate in non-Western countries, while indigenous measures may have better predictive validity
2. Providers urgently need the knowledge of indigenous psychology to solve local problesm, especially in developing countries
3. Nationalism, or anticolonialism

He does not mention yet another way in which the decolonization of mental health services can benefit global health — improving mental health care in the Western world. This book has referenced many mental health interventions originating in non-Western cultures that can be used worldwide.

Hodge (2018a) has called attention to the dramatic increase in the global refugee population in recent years. This population shares the common experiences of displacement, trauma, and the necessity of adapting to a different culture in their new countries, and many refugees are fleeing persecution based on their religious identity. All of this presents a challenge to their mental health. Hodge notes that and the fact that though religion plays an important role in the lives of many refugees, most mental health professionals have received little, if any, culturally competent training in this area. Rayes *et al.* (2021) have studied Arabic-speaking refugees, mostly Muslim, seeking mental health services in Germany and found that their faith-based coping techniques vary depending on the stage of their migration journey. During their flight, refugees reported prayer and gratitude during or at the end of their journey. Once they arrived in Germany, they faced decisions about whether to retain their faith practices in the face of reduced access to mosques and lack of cultural support. Most felt that their faith and the associated practices served as a source of comfort and reassurance throughout their mental distress. When they were asked what they would like the German mental health providers to know about their cultures or spiritual backgrounds in order to be more helpful to them, they expressed a preference for Arab-speaking professionals, a greater understanding of the trauma they had endured, and a better understanding of their culture and its traditional methods of coping. Hodge (2018b) recommends initial brief spiritual assessment using the iCaring protocol (see Chapter 7) to identify spiritual resources that refugees can use to address the problems they are currently experiencing. This can be followed by a more comprehensive spiritual assessment if it seems that spiritual issues are relevant in service provision. Pandya (2018a) studied over 4,504 refugees in 38 camps in nine different countries and found that a specially designed spirituality program reduced trauma, increased optimism, and improved mental health.

Bedi (2018) criticizes the exportation of Western notions of counseling and psychotherapy to other countries at a high rate, often without sufficient scrutiny, and even when they are inconsistent with non-Western beliefs and social values. He argues that longstanding indigenous healing practices may be more effective for "individuals who do not subscribe to the assumptions, customs, cultural principles, and culturally promoted objectives that underlie the Western practices of counseling and psychotherapy". Accepting the fact that this process is inevitable, he proposes three ways in which indigenous and Western healing methods can be integrated and recommends research on outcomes of such integration.

1. **Focusing on preexisting cultural congruence of current Western methods.** Rather than exporting a Western intervention on the basis of Western evidence, start with the cultural beliefs of a society and determine which Western psychotherapeutic interventions or theories are already most consistent and implement those.
2. **Collaboration with traditional healers as equals.** This requires further research on the viability and outcomes associated with various models of collaboration. Some have already been piloted and although they are rare, some have already proved effective. Bedi gives an example in which an African shaman was treated as a consultant for psychotherapy and a complementary provider for physical conditions to complement Western medical treatments.
3. **Using traditional healers to provide culturally congruent psychological interventions.** Western psychological interventions could be incorporated into existing indigenous healing methods and provided by lay community members under the guidance of traditional healers or by the traditional healers themselves. This alternative would have the advantage of increasing the supply of mental health care providers in under-resourced areas.

12.2 Promoting holistic definitions of mental health

Decolonizing our conceptualizations of mental health and illness involves going beyond the pathologizing orientation of the medical model to focus on health rather than illness. The World Health Organization has explored the possibility of including spiritual health in its definition of health, which currently includes physical, mental, and social dimensions (Dhar *et al.*, 2011), but has not yet formally incorporated this fourth dimension of health. The World Psychiatric Society, however, takes the position that the relevance of spirituality and religion should be central to clinical and academic psychiatry (Moreira-Almeida *et al.*, 2016). They propose (pp. 1–2) that:

1. An understanding of religion and spirituality and their relationship to the diagnosis, etiology and treatment of psychiatric disorders should be considered as essential components of both psychiatric training and continuing professional development.
2. There is a need for more research on both religion and spirituality in psychiatry, especially on their clinical applications. These studies should cover a wide diversity of cultural and geographical backgrounds.
3. The approach to religion and spirituality should be person-centered. Psychiatrists should not use their professional position for proselytizing for spiritual or secular worldviews. Psychiatrists should be expected always to respect and be sensitive to the spiritual/religious beliefs and practices of their patients, and of the families and caregivers of their patients.
4. Psychiatrists, whatever their personal beliefs, should be willing to work with leaders/members of faith communities, chaplains and pastoral workers, and others in the community, in support of the well-being of their patients, and should encourage their multidisciplinary colleagues to do likewise.
5. Psychiatrists should demonstrate awareness, respect and sensitivity to the important part that spirituality and religion play for many staff and volunteers in forming a vocation to work in the field of mental health care.
6. Psychiatrists should be knowledgeable concerning the potential for both benefit and harm of religious, spiritual, and secular worldviews and practices and be willing to share this information in a critical but impartial way with the wider community in support of the promotion of health and well-being.

These are important principles for guiding practice in this area and are echoed by other guidelines for mental health professionals.

12.3 Advancing the evidence-based research base

A number of experts have called to the inadequacy of existing research on spiritual interventions in mental health care and have drawn attention to the need for rigorous, evidence-based research on spirituality and psychotherapy (e.g., Kennedy *et al.*, 2015; Plante, 2009; Richards & Worthington, 2010). Clinical professionals engaged in research on spiritually integrated psycho-therapy would benefit from working collaboratively to conduct studies and determine best practices among theistic and other spiritual approaches. Research could begin with an investigation of the effectiveness of Plante's "Thirteen Tools" (see Chapter 8). While such collaboration is already under-way, more research is needed. Plante (2009) strongly advocates the collabora-tion of researchers with both clinicians and clerics to develop "thoughtful and sophisticated research projects":

> With some effort, researchers can work closely and collaboratively with both clinicians and clerics to develop thoughtful and sophisticated research projects. Having clerical collaborators and consultants on research teams and integrating their work into clinical protocols is an important and per-haps vital step in developing the kinds of quality research projects that are thoughtful and thus ultimately more valuable for the profession as well as for the public (p. 179).

Ee *et al.* (2020) also call for rigorous research on adjunctive approaches to mental health treatment, such as nutritional or dietary supplements (nutraceuticals), lifestyle changes, and behavior change.

12.4 Integrating spirituality into practice and training

A Pew Research Center survey found that worldwide, 84% of people identify with a religious group (2012). The religiously unaffiliated include atheists, agnostics and people who do not report identifying with any particular reli-gion. The same survey found that many of the religiously unaffiliated have some religious belief and though the survey did not ask about spirituality, it is highly probable that many had some spiritual beliefs and/or practices.

Surveys in many parts of the world have found mental health profession-als to have positive views about incorporating spirituality into psychotherapy (e.g., Vandenberghe *et al.*, 2021; Lee & Baumann, 2013; Dhar *et al.*, 2011; Charzyńska & Heszen-Celińska, 2020; Ghaderi *et al.*, 2018; Laher & Bulbulia, 2013). Oxhandler *et al.* (2015) administered a questionnaire enti-tled the Religious/Spiritually Integrated Practice Assessment Scale to licensed clinical social workers and found that while these clinicians had positive attitudes about such integration and felt able to do it, in fact they rarely did do it. The best predictors of a spiritually integrated practice were the social workers' religiosity and their prior training in the matter. In a later paper (Oxhandler *et al.*, 2018), the same data on social workers were compared to national survey data for the U.S. population. The authors found that, com-pared to the general population, the social workers were less likely to identify as Protestant or Catholic, to engage in frequent prayer, and to self-identify as religious. The social workers were, however, more likely to engage in medita-tion and to consider themselves spiritual.

Mental health professionals who have had relevant prior training are more likely to express positive attitudes about integrating spirituality into their psychotherapy practice (Oxhander *et al.*, 2015) but professional training in this area has been found lacking (e.g., Jafari, 2015; Cunha & Scorsolini-Comin, 2020; Ekşi *et al.*, 2016; Lee & Baumann, *op cit.*). Vieten *et al.* (2013) surveyed psychologists and found that though the majority agreed that psychologists should receive training in integrating psychology into their practice, the vast majority said that had received little or no training. Oman (2018) argues that courses on religion and spiritual-ity should be offered for every major public health subfield. Training in collaboration with clergy and other spiritual leaders, traditional healers, and complementary care providers is especially deficient. Richards *et al.* (2015) call for worldwide collaboration to bring spiritually oriented psy-chotherapies into the health care mainstream, pointing out that the evi-dence base for their use is still weak to non-existent and that training in the spiritual aspects of diversity is not yet adequately included in graduate education or professional continuing education opportunities. They describe a practice-based research network called Bridges that has been formed to facilitate such collaboration (https://education.byu.edu/consortium/bridges).

Though clergy typically receive some training in psychology during their studies, they can benefit from learning more about mental illness and collaboration with mental health professions. NAMI FaithNet (https://www.nami.org/Get-Involved/NAMI-FaithNet) and Mental Health Ministries (https://www.nami.org/Get-Involved/NAMI-FaithNet) are two non-profit organizations that offer clergy opportunities to learn more about supporting and referring individuals with mental illness.

12.5 Working with clergy and faith-based communities

Wong *et al.* (2017) have analyzed national survey data on religious congregations and found that close to 25% of religious congregations in the U.S. offer some type of programming to support people with mental illness. Larger and more affluent congregations and those with staff for social service or health-focused programs were more likely to provide mental health support. Heseltine-Carp & Hoskins (2020), based on a survey of UK clergy, have referred to clergy as "a frontline mental health service". Between 60 and 80% of the clergy studied reported that they regularly encountered congregants with mental health disorders and seemed effective at recognizing and referring them. They generally did not receive referrals from mental health professionals, however. These authors recommend improving spiritual training for mental health professionals and mental health training for clergy.

Schroeder (n.d.) has prepared a mental health resource and study guide for clergy and communities of faith. The main topics covered are understanding mental illness, spiritual resources for coping with mental illness, creating congregations that are supportive of the mentally ill, and more advanced training for faith leaders. DeKraal *et al.* (2011) have created a pyramid depicting the levels of services provided by community agencies and discussed the role of faith-based congregations in providing support. As Figure 12.1 shows, treatment and clinical care account for the smallest portion of mental health services and the ones in which faith communities are least likely to be involved in because of training and licensing requirements. Support services, shown in the middle of the pyramid, are more frequently used because of the financial and other kinds of instability that can result from an episode of mental illness or a chronic mental health condition. Faith communities can provide a great deal of support at this level. Such

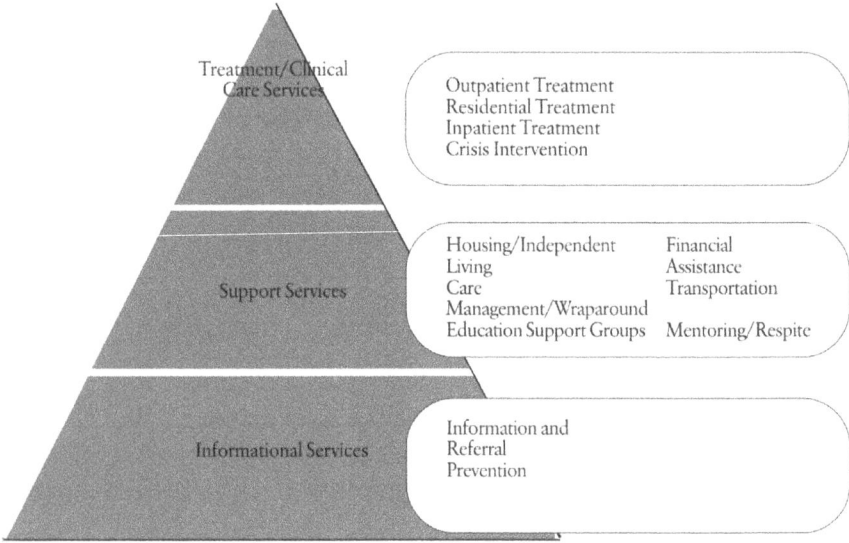

Figure 12.1.   Levels of mental health care and the potential role of faith communities.

organizations can be even more active in providing the services shown at the base of the pyramid — information, referral, and prevention.

Van Rensburg *et al.* (2014) interviewed psychiatrists and religious or spiritual advisors in South Africa and found that both groups believed that referral and collaboration between psychiatrists and spiritual professionals were important. The authors believed that the best approach would be to organize the liaison between the two types of professional into formalized referral systems or multidisciplinary teams. But since this would be difficult and logistically challenging, they suggest that the most practical approach may be to consider them as parallel systems and focus on increasing information sharing and mutual awareness between them. Overcoming the problem of stigma with regard to mental illness was considered important by both groups of professionals.

Discussion question

The World Health Organization's Mental Health Gap Action Program is an attempt to scale up (expand) mental health care in countries with a shortage of specialty mental health services by training non-specialist health care providers, or in some cases traditional healers, to implement evidence-based protocols to deliver mental health services. Some argue that this is a good solution for providing mental health care in under-resourced countries. Others oppose this strategy, arguing that it provides a poorer quality of care for the mentally ill in poorer countries. Still others see it as a form of neocolonialism in which Western culture is being imposed on non-Western countries. What is your opinion in this matter? What kind of research do you think might help to answer some of the questions that this strategy raises?

Exercise

Develop an outline for a program that would increase the awareness of the kinds of mental health resources and support that faith-based communities might be able to offer their clients.

Resources

Interfaith Network on Mental Illness: http://inmi.us/links-to-more-resources-on-faithspiritualityreligion-and-mental-health/

National Alliance for the Mentally Ill Faithnet: http://inmi.us/links-to-more-resources-on-faithspiritualityreligion-and-mental-health/

References

Abbasi, Y. (2016). As a psychiatrist I've seen how culture affect views of mental illness. *The Guardian*. Retrieved from https://www.theguardian.com/healthcare-network/views-from-the-nhs-frontline/2016/aug/08/psychiatrist-seen-culture-affects-views-mental-illness.

Abbot, S. (2007). Growth of "new media" fatwas rankles traditional Islamic establishment. *Associated Press*. Retrieved from https://azdailysun.com/lifestyles/faith-and-values/religion/growth-of-new-media-fatwas-rankles-traditional-islamic-establishment/article_518edaeb-a6cb-543c-93cf-92ac1af03f6c.html.

Abernethy, A. D., & Lancia, J. L. (1998). Religion and the psychotherapeutic relationship. Transferential and countertransferential dimensions. *Psychotherapy Practice Research, 7*(4), 281–289.

Abramowitz, J. S., & Buchholz, J. L. (2020). Spirituality/religion and obsessive-compulsive-related disorders. In D. H. Rosmarin & H. G. Koenig (Eds.), *Handbook of Spirituality, Religion, and Mental Health* (pp. 61–78). Elsevier Science & Technology.

Adams, W. Y. (1984). The first colonial empire: Egypt in Nubia, 3200–1200 BC. *Comparative Studies in Society and History, 26*(1), 36–71.

Adelson, S. L., Walker-Cometta, E., & Kalish, N. (2019). LGBT youth, mental health, and spiritual care: Psychiatric collaboration with health care chaplains. *Journal of the Academy of Child and Adolescent Psychiatry, 58*(7), 651–655.

Ainsworth, M. D. (1964). Patterns of attachment behavior shown by the infant in interaction with his mother. *Merrill-Palmer Quarterly of Behavior and Development, 10*(1), 51–58.

Altemeyer, B., & Hunsberger, B. E. (1992). Authoritarianism, religious fundamentalism, quest, and prejudice. *International Journal for the Psychology of Religion, 2*(2), 113–133.

Al'Uqdah, S. N., Hamit, S., & Scott, S. (2019). African American Muslims: Intersectionality and cultural competence. *Counseling and Values, 64*(2), 130–147.

American Association for Marriage and Family Therapy. (2015). American Association for Marriage and Family Therapy Code of Ethics. *American Association for Marriage and Family Therapy (AAMFT)*. Retrieved from https://www.aamft.org/Legal_Ethics/Code_of_Ethics.aspx.

American Civil Liberties Union. (n.d.). Using religion to discriminate. *American Civil Liberties Union*. Retrieved from https://www.aclu.org/issues/religious-liberty/using-religion-discriminate/end-use-religion-discriminate.

American Counseling Association. (2009). Competencies for addressing spiritual and religious issues in counseling. *American Counseling Association*. Retrieved from https://www.counseling.org/docs/default-source/competencies/competencies-for-addressing-spiritual-and-religious-issues-in-counseling.pdf?sfvrsn=aad7c2c_10.

American Counseling Association. (2014). American Counseling Association Code of Ethics. *American Counseling Association*. Retrieved from https://www.counseling.org/docs/default-source/default-document-library/2014-code-of-ethics-finaladdress.pdf?sfvrsn=96b532c_2.

American Psychiatric Association. (2013a). *The Principles of Medical Ethics with Annotations Especially Applicable to Psychiatry*. American Psychiatric Association.

American Psychiatric Association. (2013b). *Diagnostic and Statistical Manual of Mental Disorders* (5th ed.). American Psychiatric Association.

American Psychiatric Association. (2018). What is mental illness? *American Psychiatric Association*. Retrieved from https://www.psychiatry.org/patients-families/what-is-mental-illness.

American Psychiatric Association (2021). Resource document on ethics at the interface of religion, spirituality, and psychiatric practice. *American Psychiatric Association*. Retrieved from https://psychnews.psychiatryonline.org/doi/10.1176/appi.pn.2021.2.22.

American Psychological Association. (2017). Ethical principles of psychologists and code of conduct. *American Psychological Association*. Retrieved from https://www.apa.org/ethics/code.

Anandarajah, G., & Hight, E. (2001). Spirituality and medical practice: Using the HOPE questions as a practical tool for spiritual assessment. *American Family Physician, 63*(1), 81–89.

André, C. (2017). Evolving story: Trepanation and self-trepanation to enhance brain function. *Arquivos de Neuro-psiquiatria, 75*(5), 307–313.

Andrews, C. R., & Marotta, S. A. (2005). Spirituality and coping among grieving children: A preliminary study. *Counseling and Values, 50*(1), 38–50.

Antonelli, M., Barbieri, G., & Donelli, D. (2019). Effects of forest bathing (shinrin-yoku) on levels of cortisol as a stress biomarker: a systematic review and meta-analysis. *International Journal of Biometeorology, 63*(8), 1117–1134.

Arain, M., Haque, M., Johal, L., Mathur, P., Nel, W., Rais, A., Sandhu, R., & Sharma, S. (2013). Maturation of the adolescent brain. *Neuropsychiatric Disease and Treatment, 9*, 449–461.

Attum, B., Hafiz, S., Malik, A., & Shamoon, Z. (2021). *Cultural Competence in the Care of Muslim Patients and their Families.* StatPearls Publishing.

Baek, H.-J. (2002). A comparative study of moral development of Korean and British children. *Journal of Moral Education, 31*(4), 373–391.

Bandura, A. (1997). *Self-Efficacy: The Exercise of Control.* W. H. Freeman and Company.

Bankson, M. Z. (1999). *The Call to the Soul.* Augsburg Fortress Publishing.

Barnett, J. E., & Johnson, W. B. (2011). Integrating spirituality and religion into psychotherapy: Persistent dilemmas, ethical issues, and a proposed decision-making process. *Ethics & Behavior, 2*(2), 147–165.

Barrera, R. L., Zeno, D., Bush, A. L., Barber, C. R., & Stanley, M. A. (2012). Integrating religion and spirituality into treatment for late-life anxiety: Three case studies. *Cognitive and Behavioral Practice, 19*(2), 346–358.

Barsky, A. E. (2019). Ethics alive! Religious freedom and social work: Ethics of referring clients. *The New Social Worker.* Retrieved from https://www.socialworker.com/feature-articles/ethics-articles/ethics-alive-religious-freedom-and-social-work-ethics-of-referring-clients/.

Barsky, A. E. (2020). Sexuality- and gender-inclusive genograms: Avoiding heteronormativity and cisnormativity. *Journal of Social Work Education,* DOI: 10.1080/10437797.2020.1852637.

Baumrind, D. (2013). Authoritative parenting revisited: History and current status. In R. E. Larzelere, A. Sheffield, & A. W. Harris (Eds.), *Authoritative Parenting: Synthesizing Nurturance and Discipline for Optimal Child Development* (pp. 11–34). American Psychological Association.

Bayne, H. B., & Tylsova, M. (2019). Understanding and incorporating God representations within counseling. *Counseling and Values, 64*(2), 148–167.

Beck, R. A., & McDonald, A. (2004). Attachment to God: The Attachment to God Inventory, tests of working model correspondence, and an exploration of faith group differences. *Journal of Psychology & Theology, 32*(2), 92–103.

Bedi, R. P. (2018). Racial, ethnic, cultural, and national disparities in counseling and psychotherapy outcome are inevitable but eliminating global mental health disparities with indigenous healing is not. *Archives of Scientific Psychology*, *6*(1), 96–104.

Bell, D. (1974). *The Coming of Post-Industrial Society*. Colophon Books.

Bernstein, L. (2021). Addiction treatment had failed. Could brain surgery save him? *The Washington Post*. Retrieved from https://www.washingtonpost.com/health/2021/06/18/deep-brain-stimulation-addiction/.

Berry, J. W., Worthington, E. L., Jr., & O'Connor, L. E. (2003). Altruism and the structure of virtue: Preferences and practices. Presented at *Works of Love: Religious and Scientific Approaches to Altruism*. Metanexus Institute.

Bettelheim, B. (1975). *The Uses of Enchantment*. Vintage Books.

Bilich, M., Bonfiglio, S., & Carlson, S. (2000). *Shared Grace: Therapists and Clergy Working Together*. Routledge.

Blanton, P. G. (2019). *Contemplation and Counseling: An Integrative Model for Practitioners*. IVP Academic.

BMJ. (2000). Doctors warn of the dangers of trepanning. *BMJ: British Medical Journal*, *320*(7235), 602.

Boas, F. (1887). Museums of ethnology and their classification. *Science*, *9*(228), 587–589.

Bojuwoye, O. (2005). Traditional healing practices in Southern Africa: Ancestral spirits, ritual ceremonies, and holistic healing. In R. Moodley & W. West (Eds.), *Integrating Traditional Healing Practices into Counseling and Psychotherapy* (pp. 61–72). SAGE Publications.

Bothwell, A. P. X. (2019). International Standards for Protection of Religious Freedom. *Annual Survey of International and Comparative Law*, *23*(1), 49–77.

Bowlby, J. (1983). *Attachment: Attachment and Loss Volume One* (2nd ed.). Basic Books.

Boynton, H. M., & Mellan, C. (2021). Co-creating authentic sacred therapeutic space: A spiritually sensitive framework for counseling children. *Religions*, *12*(7), 524.

Bożek, A., Nowak, P. F., & Blukacz, M. (2020). The relationship between spirituality, health-related behavior, and psychological well-being. *Frontiers in Psychology*, *11*, 1997.

Brisch, K. H. (2014). *Treating Attachment Disorders: From Theory to Therapy* (2nd ed.). Guilford Press.

Bromberg, W. (1975). *From Shaman to Psychotherapist: A History of the Treatment of Mental Illness* (4th ed.). Regnery.

Bromley, D. (2016). Santa Muerte as emerging dangerous religion?. *Religions*, *7*(6), 65.

Bruchhausen, W. (2018). Medicalized healing in East Africa. In D. Lüddekens & M. Schrimp (Eds.), *Medicine — Religion — Spirituality: Global Perspectives on Traditional, Complementary, and Alternative Healing* (pp. 23–55). Transcript Verlag.

Buchtel, E. E. (2014). Cultural sensitivity or cultural stereotyping? Positive and negative effects of a cultural psychology class. *International Journal of Intercultural Relations, 39*(March), 40–52.

Burch-Brown, J., & Baker, W. (2016). Religion and reducing prejudice. *Group Processes and Intergroup Relations, 19*(6), 784–807.

Burger, J. R., & Fristoe, T. S. (2018). Hunter-gatherer populations inform modern ecology. *Proceedings of the National Academy of Sciences of the United States of America, 115*(6), 1137–1139.

Burston, D. (1998). *The Wing of Madness: The Life and Work of R.D. Laing.* Harvard University Press.

Busch, H., Jofer, J., Šolcová, I. P., & Tavel, P. (2018). Generativity affects fear of death through ego integrity in German, Czech, and Cameroonian older adults. *Archives of Gerontology and Geriatrics, 77*(July-August), 89–95.

Butler, R. N. (1963). Life review: An interpretation of reminiscence in the aged. *Psychiatry, 26*(1), 65–76.

Callahan, A. M. (2017). *Spirituality and Hospice Social Work.* Columbia University Press.

Cameron, J. (1992). *The Artist's Way.* TarcherPerigee.

Campbell, J. (2020). *The Hero with A Thousand Faces* (3rd ed.). Joseph Campbell Foundation.

Canda, E. R., & Furman, L. D. (2010). *Spiritual Diversity in Social Work Practice: The Heart of Helping.* Oxford University Press.

Canda, E. R., Moon, J., & Kim, K. M. (2017). *Korean Social Welfare's Approach to Spiritual Diversity.* Routledge.

Caplan, G., Caplan, R. B., & Erchul, W. P. (1995). A contemporary view of mental health consultation: Comments on "types of mental health consultation" by Gerald Caplan. *Journal of Educational and Psychological Consultation, 6*(1), 23–30.

Carle, R. (2018). Islamically integrated psychotherapy. *Journal of Religion and Health, 58,* 541–547.

Cashwell, C. S., Bentley, P. B., & Yarborough, P. (2007). The only way out is through: The perils of spiritual bypass. *Counseling and Values, 51*(2), 139–148.

Cassidy, J. (1999). The nature of a child's ties. In J. Cassidy & P. R. Shaver (Eds.), *Handbook of Attachment: Theory, Research and Clinical Applications* (pp. 3–20). Guilford Press.

Çetintaş, S., & Ekşi, H. (2020). Spiritually oriented couple, marriage, and family therapies. *Spiritual Psychology and Counseling, 5*(1), 7–24.

Chakkarath, P. (2013). Indian thoughts on human psychological development. In G. Misra (Ed.), *Psychology and Psychoanalysis* (pp. 167–190). Munshiram Manoharlal Publishers.

Charzyńska, E., & Heszen-Celińska, I. (2020). Spirituality and mental health care in a religiously homogeneous country: Definitions, opinions, and practices among Polish mental health professionals. *Journal of Religion and Health, 59*, 113–134.

Clarke, P. B., Giordano, A. L., Cashwell, C. S., & Lewis, T. F. (2013). The straight path to healing: Using motivational interviewing to address spiritual bypass. *Journal of Counseling and Development, 91*(1), 87–94.

Cleveland Council on World Affairs. (2014). Economic and Social Council Background Guide. Cleveland Council on World Affairs. *Cleveland Council on World Affairs.* Retrieved from https://www.ccwa.org/wp-content/uploads/2014/03/FINAL-ECOSOC-Background-Guide.pdf.

Cohen, S. (1973). *Folk Devils and Moral Panics.* Paladin.

Coholic, D. (2010). *Arts Activities for Children and Young People in Need.* Jessica Kingsley Publishers.

Coles, R. (1990). *The Spiritual Life of Children.* Houghton Mifflin.

Compton, W. (2012). *Eastern Psychology.* CreateSpace.

Connery, H. S., & Devido, J. (2020). Spirituality/religion and substance use disorders. In D. H. Rosmarin & H. G. Koenig (Eds.), *Handbook of Spirituality, Religion, and Mental Health* (pp. 119–138). Elsevier Science & Technology.

Corbett, L. (2011). *The Sacred Cauldron: Psychotherapy as a Spiritual Practice.* Chiron Publications.

Cox, D., & Jones, R. P. (2017). America's changing religious identity. *Public Religion Research Institute (PRRI).* Retrieved from https://www.prri.org/research/american-religious-landscape-christian-religiously-unaffiliated/.

Coyle, N. (2004). The existential slap — a crisis of disclosure. *International Journal of Palliative Nursing, 10*(11), 520.

Crenshaw, K. W. (1989). Demarginalizing the intersection of race and sex: A Black Feminist critique of antidiscrimination doctrine, Feminist theory, and antiracist politics. *University of Chicago Legal Forum, 1989*(1), 139–167.

Crenshaw, K. W. (2017). *On Intersectionality: Selected Writings.* The New Press.

Crisp, B. R. (2014). *Social Work and Faith-Based Organizations.* Routledge.

Cross, T. L., Bazron, B. J., Dennis, K. W., & Isaacs, M. R. (1989). *Towards a Culturally Competent System of Care: A Monograph on Effective Services for Minority Children Who Are Severely Emotionally Disturbed.* Georgetown University Child Development Center.

Crowley, N. (2006). Psychosis or spiritual emergence. *Royal College of Psychiatrists*. Retrieved from https://www.rcpsych.ac.uk/docs/default-source/members/sigs/spirituality-spsig/spirituality-special-interest-group-publications-nicki-crowley-psychosis-or-spiritual-emergence.pdf?sfvrsn=5685d4c1_2.

Cumming, E., & Henry, W. (1961). *Growing Old: The Process of Disengagement*. Basic Books.

Cunha, V. F., & Scorsolini-Comin, F. (2020). Brazilian psychotherapists and the dimension of religiosity/spirituality. *Counseling and Psychotherapy Research*, *21*(2), 281–289.

Curry, J. R. (2009). Examining client spiritual history and the construction of meaning: The use of spiritual timelines in counseling. *Journal of Creativity in Mental Health*, *4*(2), 113–123.

Curtis, J. B. *et al.* (2017). Collaboration between clergy and mental health professionals in post-disaster contexts: Lessons from the Big Branch mine disaster. *Spirituality in Clinical Practice*, *4*(3), 193–204.

Czikszentmihalyi, M. (2008). *Flow: The Psychology of Optimal Experience*. Harper Perennial Modern Classics.

Dana, D. A. (2018). *The Polyvagal Theory in Therapy: Engaging the Rhythm of Regulation*. W.W. Norton.

Day, A. (2020). Towards increasing diversity in the study of religion. *Religion*, *50*(1), 45–52.

DeKraal, M. B., Billling, D. J., Shank, N., & Tomkins, A. J. (2011). Faith-based organizations in a system of behavioral health care. *Journal of Psychology and Theology*, *39*(3), 255–267.

Dempsey, K., Butler, S. K., & Gaither, L. (2016). Black churches and mental health professionals. Can this collaboration work? *Journal of Black Studies*, *47*(1), 73–87.

de Rios, M. D. (2002). What we can learn from shamanic healing: Brief psychotherapy with Latino immigrant clients. *American Journal of Public Health*, *92*(10), 1576–1581.

Dhar, N., Chaturvedi, S. K., & Nandan, D. (2011). Spiritual health scale 2011: Defining and measuring 4th dimension of health. *Indian Journal of Community Medicine*, *36*(4), 275–282.

Dietrich, A. (2004). Neurocognitive mechanisms underlying the experience of flow. *Consciousness and Cognition*, *13*(4), 746–761.

Dollahite, D. C. (1998). Origins and highlights of the special issue on fathering, faith, and spirituality. *Journal of Men's Studies*, *7*, 1–2.

Doostdar, A. (2019). Impossible occultists: Practice and participation in an Islamic tradition. *American Ethnologist*, *46*(2), 178–189.

Dubuisson, D. (2007). *The Western Construction of Religion: Myths, Knowledge, and Ideology*. Johns Hopkins University Press.

Duclow, D. F. (2002). William James, mind-cure, and the religion of healthy-mindedness. *Journal of Religion and Health*, *41*(1), 45–56.

Dudley, J. R. (2016). *Spirituality Matters in Social Work*. Routledge.

Durkheim, E., & Swain, W. (1916). The elementary forms of religious life. *American Journal of Nursing*, *16*(12), 1248.

Earlywine, M., Ueno, L. F., Mian, M. M., & Altman, B. R. (2021). Cannabis-induced oceanic boundlessness. *Journal of Psychopharmacology*, *35*(7), 841–847.

Edelman, G. M. (2004). *Wider than the Sky*. Yale University Press.

Ee, C., Lake, J., Firth, J., Hargraves, F., de Manincor, M., Meade, T., Marx, W., & Sarris, J. (2020). An integrative collaborative care model for people with mental illness and physical comorbidities. *International Journal of Health Systems*, *14*(1), 83.

Egan, J. (2020). Covid hikikomori: An Ode to those who might never emerge from lockdown. *Forbes*. Retrieved from https://www.forbes.com/sites/johnegan/2020/11/18/covid-hikikomori-an-ode-to-those-who-will-never-emerge-from-lockdown/?sh=12bc0dbe73bf.

Ekşi, H., Takmaz, Z., & Kardaş, S. (2016). Spirituality in psychotherapy settings: A phenomenological inquiry into the experiences of Turkish health professionals. *Spiritual Psychology and Counseling*, *1*(1), 89–108.

Eliade, M. (2020). *Shamanism: Archaic Techniques of Ecstasy*. Princeton University Press.

Ellis, E. E., Yilanli, M., & Saabadi, A. (1921). *Reactive Attachment Disorder*. StatPearls.

Emmons, R. A., & Paloutzian, R. F. (2003). The psychology of religion. *Annual Review of Psychology*, *54*, 377–402.

Enroth, R. M. (1992). *Churches that Abuse*. Zondevan.

Epstein, G. M. (2009). *Good without God*. HarperCollins.

Erikson, E. H. (1980). *Identity and the Life Cycle*. W.W. Norton.

Erikson, E. H., & Erickson, J. M. (1998). *The Life Cycle Completed (Extended Version)*. W.W. Norton.

Fadiman, A. (1998). *The Spirit Catches You and You Fall Down*. Farrar, Straus and Giroux.

Feiler, B. (2021). *Life Is in the Transitions: Mastering Change at Any Age*. Penguin Books.

Ferguson, M. A., Schaper, F. L. W. V. J., Cohen, A., Siddiqi, S., Merrill, S. M., Nielsen, J. A., Grafman, J., Urgesi, C., Fabbro, F., & Fox, M. D. (2021). A neural circuit for spirituality and religiosity derived from patients with brain lesions. *Biological Psychiatry*, *91*(4), 380–388.

Fincher, S. F. (2010). *Creating Mandalas*. Shambhala.

Fisher, J. (2011). The four domains model: Connecting spirituality, health, and wellbeing. *Religions, 2*(1), 17–28.

Fitzgerald, T. (2007). *Discourse on Civility and Barbarity*. Oxford University Press.

Fortune, M. M., & Enger, C. G. (2005). Violence against women and the role of religion. *National Online Resource Center on Violence Against Woman*. Retrieved from https://vawnet.org/sites/default/files/materials/files/2016-09/AR_VAWReligion_0.pdf.

Fowler, J. W. (1995). *Stages of Faith: The Psychology of Human Development and the Quest for Meaning*. HarperCollins.

Fox, J. (2020). *Thou Shalt Have No Other Gods before Me*. Cambridge University Press.

Frankl, V. E. (1967). Logotherapy and existentialism. *Psychotherapy: Theory, Research & Practice, 4*(3), 138–142.

Freire, J., Moliero, C., Rosmarin, D. H., & Freire, M. (2019). A call for collaboration: Perception of religious and spiritual leaders on mental health (A Portuguese sample). *Journal of Spirituality in Mental Health, 21*(1), 55–75.

Freud, S. (1919). *Totem and Taboo*. Beacon Press.

Fuller, R. C. (2017). Secular spirituality. In P. Zuckerman & J. R. Shook (Eds.), *The Oxford Handbook of Secularism* (pp. 571–586). Oxford University Press.

Gecewicz, C. (2018). 'New Age' beliefs common among both religious and nonreligious Americans. *Pew Research Center*. Retrieved from https://www.pewresearch.org/fact-tank/2018/10/01/new-age-beliefs-common-among-both-religious-and-nonreligious-americans/.

Gendlin, E. T. (1982). *Focusing*. Bantam.

Ghaderi, A., Tabatabaei, S. M., Nedjat, S., Javadi, M., & Larijani, B. (2018). Explanatory definition of the concept of spiritual health: a qualitative study in Iran. *Journal of Medical Ethics in the History of Medicine, 11*(3), 1–7.

Ghorbani, N., Watson, P. J., Geranmayepour, S., & Chen, Z. (2014). Measuring Muslim spirituality: Relationships of Muslim experiential religiousness with religious and psychological adjustments in Iran. *Journal of Muslim Mental Health, 8*(1), 77–94.

Gilligan, C. (1982). *In a Different Voice*. Harvard University Press.

Gomes, J. F. (2013). Religious diversity, intolerance, and civil conflict. *Universidad Carlos III de Madrid*. Retrieved from https://core.ac.uk/download/pdf/29404273.pdf.

Gone, J. P. (2008). Introduction: Mental health discourse as Western cultural proselytization. *Ethos, 36*(3), 310–315.

Gonzales, P. (2012). Calling our spirits back.: Indigenous ways of diagnosing and treating soul sickness. *Fourth World Journal, 11*(2), 25–59.

Goulet, N. (2011). Postcolonialism and the study of religion: Dissecting orientalism, nationalism, and gender using postcolonial theory. *Religion Compass, 5*(10), 631–637.

Grafman, J., Cristofori, I., Zhong, W., & Bulbulia, J. (2020). The neural basis of religious cognition. *Current Directions in Psychological Science, 29*(2), 126–133.

Graham, M. (2005). Maat: An African-centered paradigm for psychological and spiritual healing. In R. Moodley & W. West (Eds.), *Integrating Traditional Healing Practices into Counseling and Psychotherapy* (pp. 210–220). Thousand Oaks.

Gregg, G. S. (2005). *The Middle East: A Cultural Psychology*. Oxford University Press.

Gregory, W. H., & Harper, K. W. (2001). The Ntu approach to health and healing. *Journal of Black Psychology, 27*(3), 304–320.

Griffith, J. L. (2012). Psychotherapy, religion, and spirituality. In R. D. Alarcon & J. B. Frank (Eds.), *The Psychotherapy of Hope* (pp. 311–325). Johns Hopkins University Press.

Grof, C., & Grof, S. (1986). Spiritual emergency: The understanding and treatment of transpersonal crises. *ReVISION, 8*(2), 7–20.

Grubbs, J. B., & Grant, J. T. (2020). Spirituality/religion and behavioral addictions. In D. H. Rosmarin & H. G. Koenig (Eds.), *Handbook of Spirituality, Religion, and Mental Health* (pp. 139–157). Elsevier Science & Technology.

Hagen, L. (2002). Taoism and psychology. In R. P. Olson (Ed.), *Religious Theories of Personality and Psychotherapy: East Meets West* (pp. 141–210). Routledge.

Harner, M. (1990). *The Way of the Shaman*. HarperOne.

Harris, K. P., Rock, A. J., & Clark, G. I. (2020). Defining spiritual emergency: A content validity study. *Journal of Transpersonal Psychology, 52*(1), 113–141.

Harrison, G. P. (2016). Why no one should ever use the word "cult". *Psychology Today*. Retrieved from https://www.psychologytoday.com/us/blog/about-thinking/201607/why-no-one-should-ever-use-the-word-cult.

Hathaway, W. L., & Ripley, J. S. (2009). Ethical concerns around spirituality and clinical practice. In J. D. Aten & M. M. Leach (Eds.), *Spirituality and the Therapeutic Process: A Comprehensive Resource from Intake to Termination* (pp. 25–52). American Psychological Association.

Hayes, S. C., & Smith, S. (2005). *Get Out of Your Mind and Into Your Life: The New Acceptance and Commitment Therapy*. New Harbinger.

Helderman, I. (2019). *Prescribing the Dharma: Buddhist Traditions and Defining Religion*. University of North Carolina Press.

Heseltine-Carp, W., & Hoskins, M. (2020). Clergy as a frontline mental health service: A UK survey of medical practitioners and clergy. *General Psychiatry*, *33*(6), e100229.

Hill, P. C., Pargament, K. I., McCullough, M. E., Swyers, J. P., & Larson, D. B. (2001). Conceptualizing religion and spirituality: Points of commonality, points of departure. *Journal for Theory of Social Behavior*, *30*(1), 51–77.

Hissan, A. (2007). Transcendent reality: An Islamic perspective. *Katib*. Retrieved from https://katib.wordpress.com/2007/05/03/transcendence-reality/.

Hoare, C. H. (2002). *Erikson on Development in Adulthood: New Insights from the Unpublished Papers*. Oxford University Press.

Hodapp, B., & Zwingmann, C. (2019). Religiosity/spirituality and mental health: A meta-analysis of studies from the German-speaking area. *Journal of Religion and Health*, *58*(6), 1970–1988.

Hodge, D. R. (2000). Spiritual ecomaps: A new diagrammatic tool for assessing marital and family spirituality. *Journal of Marital and Family Therapy*, *26*(2), 217–228.

Hodge, D. R. (2001). Spiritual genograms: A generational approach to assessing spirituality. *Families in Society: The Journal of Contemporary Human Services*, *82*(1), 35–48.

Hodge, D. R. (2005a). Spiritual lifemaps: A client-centered pictorial instrument for spiritual assessment, planning, and intervention. *Social Work*, *50*(1), 77–87.

Hodge, D. R. (2005b). Spiritual ecograms: A new assessment instrument for identifying clients' strengths in space and across time. *Families in Society: The Journal of Contemporary Human Services*, *82*(2), 287–296.

Hodge, D. R. (2007). The spiritual competence scale: A new instrument for assessing spiritual competence at the programmatic level. *Research on Social Work Practice*, *17*(2), 287–295.

Hodge, D. R., & Holtrop, C. R. (2008). Spiritual assessment: A review of complementary assessment models. In B. Hugen & T. L. Scales (Eds.), *Christianity and Social Work: Readings on the Integration of Christian Faith and Social Work Practice* (pp. 217–238). North American Association of Christians in Social Work.

Hodge, D. R., Bonifas, E., & Chou, R. (2010). Spirituality and older adults: Ethical guidelines to enhance service provision in social work practice. *Advances in Social Work*, *11*(1), 1–16.

Hodge, D. R. (2015). *Spiritual Assessment in Social Work and Mental Health Practice*. Columbia University Press.

Hodge, D. R. (2018a). Administering spiritual assessments with refugees: An overview of conceptually distinct assessment options. *Journal of Religious Studies*, 33(3), 479–499.

Hodge, D. R. (2018b). Spiritual competence: What it is, why it is necessary, and how to develop it. *Journal of Ethnic and Cultural Diversity in Social Work*, 27(2), 124–139.

Horiguchi, S. (2014). Hikikomori: Adolescence without end. *Social Science Japan Journal*, 18(1), 138–141.

Horovitz, E. G. (2017). *Spiritual Art Therapy: An Alternate Path*. Charles C. Thomas.

Horowitz, J. (2021). Pope widens church law to target sexual abuse of adults by priests and laity. *The New York Times*. Retrieved from https://www.nytimes.com/2021/06/01/world/europe/vatican-priests-sexual-abuse.html.

Hoskins, D., & Platt, D. (2021). Building a collaborative framework: a qualitative study of therapists collaborating with Curanderxs. *The Journal of Mental Health Training, Education, and Practice*, DOI: 10.1108/JMHTEP-05-2021-0043.

Houtman, D., & Meyer, B. (2013). Things: Religion and the question of materiality. *Fordham Scholarship Online*. Retrieved from https://fordham.universitypressscholarship.com/view/10.5422/fordham/9780823239450.001.0001/upso-9780823239450-chapter-1.

Howe, D., & Fearnley, S. (1999). Disorders of attachment and attachment therapy. *Adoption and Fostering*, 23(2), 19–30.

Hughes, M. E., Waite, L. J., Hawkley, L. C., & Caccioppo, J. T. (2004). A short scale for measuring loneliness in large surveys. *Research on Aging*, 26(6), 655–672.

Huguelet, P. (2020). Spirituality, religion, and psychotic disorders. In D. H. Rosmarin & H. G. Koenig (Eds.), *Handbook of Spirituality, Religion, and Mental Health* (pp. 79–97). Elsevier Science & Technology.

Human Rights Watch. (2017). Saudi Arabia: Religion Textbooks Promote Intolerance. *Human Rights Watch*. Retrieved from https://www.hrw.org/news/2017/09/13/saudi-arabia-religion-textbooks-promote-intolerance.

Huxley, A. (1945). *The Perennial Philosophy*. Harper & Brothers.

Introvigne, M. (2000). Moral panics and anti-cult terrorism in Western Europe. *Terrorism and Political Violence*, 12(1), 47–59.

Jackson, L. J., White, C. R., O'Brien, K., DiLorenzo, P., Cathcart, E., Wolf, M., Bruskas, D., Pecora, P. J., Nix-Early, V., & Cabrera, J. (2010). Exploring spirituality among youth in foster care: findings from the Casey Field Office mental health study. *Child and Family Social Work*, 1(5), 100–107.

Jacob, K. S. (2015). Recovery model of mental illness: A complementary approach to psychiatric care. *Indian Journal of Psychological Medicine*, 37(Apr-Jun), 117–119.

Jafari, S. (2015). Religion and spirituality within counselling/clinical psychology training programmes: a systematic review. *British Journal of Guidance and Counseling, 44*(3), 257–267.

James, W. (1890). *The Principles of Psychology.* Henry Holt & Company.

James, W. (1902). *The Varieties of Religious Experience: A Study in Human Nature, Being the Gifford Lectures on Natural Religion Delivered at Edinburgh in 1901–1902.* Longmans, Green & Co.

Jenkins, P. (1988). *Moral Panic Changing Concepts of the Child Molester in Modern America.* Yale University Press.

Johansen, B. (2003). *Indigenous People and Environmental Issues.* Greenwood Press.

Joint Public Issues Team. (n.d.). Religious Persecution. *Joint Public Issues Team.* Retrieved from http://www.jointpublicissues.org.uk/issues/religious-persecution/.

Joubert, N. (2018). *Psychology and Psychotherapy in the Perspective of Christian Anthropology.* Cambridge Scholars Publishing.

Jung, C. G. (1964). *Man and His Symbols.* Aldous Books.

Jung, C. G. (1972). *Two Essays on Analytical Psychology* (2nd ed.). Princeton University Press.

Jung, C. G. (2001). *Modern Man in Search of a Soul.* Routledge.

Kakar, S. (2020). The psychology of riots: The dark side of religious identity is communal identity, characterised by intolerance and potential for violence. *The Times of India.* Retrieved from https://timesofindia.indiatimes.com/blogs/toi-edit-page/the-psychology-of-riots-communalism-is-the-dark-side-of-religious-identity-beware-demagogues-availing-our-group-narcissism/.

Kalin, M., & Siddiqui, N. (2014). Religious authority and the promotion of sectarian tolerance in Pakistan. *United States Institute of Peace.* Retrieved from https://www.usip.org/sites/default/files/SR354_Religious-Authority-and-the-Promotion-of-Sectarian-Tolerance-in-Pakistan.pdf.

Kállai, I., & Kéri, S. (2020). Religious-spiritual crisis or psychosis? The impact of basic symptoms in the differentiation of prepsychotic states. *Psychiatria Hungarica, 35*(2), 102–110.

Karpov, V., & Lisovskaya, E. (2007). Religious intolerance among Orthodox Christians and Muslims in Russia. *The National Council for Eurasian and East European Research.* Retrieved from https://www.ucis.pitt.edu/nceeer/2007_820-11g_Karpov.pdf.

Kaselionyte, J., & Gumley, A. (2019). Psychosis or spiritual emergency? A Foucauldian discourse analysis of case reports of extreme mental states in the context of meditation. *Transcultural Psychiatry, 56*(5), 1094–1115.

Keller, R. C. (2007). *Colonial Madness: Psychiatry in French North Africa*. University of Chicago Press.

Kennedy, G. A., Macnab, F. A., & Ross, J. J. (2015). *The Effectiveness of Spiritual/ Religious Interventions in Psychotherapy and Counselling: A Review of the Recent Literature*. The Psychotherapy and Counselling Federation of Australia.

Kennedy, M. (2010). India's mentally ill turn to faith, not medicine. *National Public Radio*. Retrieved from https://www.npr.org/templates/story/story.php?storyId=126143778.

Keskínoğlu, M., & Ekşí, H. (2019). Islamic spiritual counseling techniques. *Spiritual Psychology and Counseling*, *4*(3), 333–350.

Kim, U., & Berry, J. W. (Eds.). (1993). *Indigenous Psychologies: Research and Experience in Cultural Context*. SAGE Publications.

Kim-Prieto, C. (2014a). *Religion and Spirituality Across Cultures*. Springer.

Kim-Prieto, C. (2014b). Introduction: Positive Psychology of Religion Across Traditions and Beliefs. In C. Kim-Prieto (Ed.), *Religion and Spirituality Across Cultures* (pp. 1–18). Springer.

Kingsbury, K., & Chesnut, R. A. (2020). Holy death in the time of coronavirus: Santa Muerte, the salubrious saint. *International Journal of Latin American Religions*, *4*, 194–217.

Knabb, J. K. (2016). *Faith-Based ACT for Christian Clients*. Routledge.

Koch, C. (2020). What near-death experiences reveal about the brain. *Scientific American*, *322*(6), 70–75.

Koenig, H. G., George, L. K., & Tius, P. (2004). Religion, spirituality, and health in medically hospitalized older patients. *Journal of the American Geriatrics Society*, *52*(4), 554–562.

Koenig, H. G. (2005). *Faith and Mental Health: Religious Resources for Healing*. Templeton.

Koenig, H. G., Peteet, J. R., & VanderWeele, T. J. (2020). Religion and psychiatry: clinical applications. *BJPsych Advances*, *26*(5), 273–281.

Koetschet, P. (2016). Experiencing madness: Mental patients in medieval Arabo-Islamic medicine. In G. Petridou & C. Thumiger (Eds.), *Homo Patiens: Approaches to the Patient in the Ancient World* (pp. 224–244). Brill.

Kohlberg, L., & Kramer, R. (1969). Continuities and discontinuities in childhood and adult moral development. *Human Development*, *12*, 93–120.

Kohlberg, L. (1984). *The Psychology of Moral Development: The Nature and Validity of Moral Stages (Essays on Moral Development, Volume 2)*. Harper & Row.

Koltko-Rivera, M. E. (2006). Rediscovering the later version of Maslow's hierarchy of needs: Self-transcendence and opportunities for theory, research, and unification. *Review of General Psychology*, *10*(4), 302–317.

Kpobi, L. N. A., & Swartz, L. (2019). Muslim traditional healers in Accra, Ghana: Beliefs about and treatment of mental disorders. *Journal of Religion and Health*, *58*, 833–846.

Kübler-Ross, E., & Kessler, D. (2005). *On Grief & Grieving*. Scribner.

Kübler-Ross, E. (2011). *On Death & Dying*. Scribner.

Kumar, S., & Shrivastava, R. (2000). Diagnosing mental illnesses by pulse examination in ancient India. *American Journal of Psychiatry*, *157*(3), 450.

Kushi, K. (2018). Key findings on the global rise in religious restrictions. *Pew Research Center*. Retrieved from https://www.pewresearch.org/fact-tank/2018/06/21/key-findings-on-the-global-rise-in-religious-restrictions/.

Laher, S., & Bulbulia, T. (2013). Exploring the role of Islam in perceptions of mental illness in a sample of Muslim psychiatrists based in Johannesburg. *South African Journal of Psychiatry*, *19*(2), 52–54.

Land, H. (2015). *Spirituality, Religion, and Faith in Psychotherapy*. Lyceum Books.

Lannert, J. L. (1991). Resistance and countertransference issues with spiritual and religious clients. *Journal of Humanistic Psychology*, *31*(4), 68–76.

Lee, E., & Baumann, K. (2013). German psychiatrists' observation and interpretation of religiosity/spirituality. *Evidence-Based Complementary and Alternative Medicine*, *2013*, 280168.

Lee, J. H. (2019). Integration of spirituality into the strengths-based social work practice: A transpersonal approach to the strengths perspective. *Journal of Sociology and Social Work*, *7*(2), 25–35.

Lewis, M. E., Hartwell, E. E., & Myhra, L. L. (2018). Decolonizing mental health services for indigenous clients: A training program for mental health professionals. *American Journal of Community Psychology*, *62*(3–4), 330–339.

Lifton, R. J. (2019). *Losing Reality: On Cults, Cultism, and the Mindset of Political and Religious Zealotry*. The New Press.

Liht, J., Conway, L. G. I., Savage, S., White, W., & O'Neill, K. A. (2011). Religious fundamentalism: An empirically derived construct and measurement scale. *Archive for the Psychology of Religion*, *33*, 1–25.

Linzer, N. (2006). Spirituality and ethics in long-term care. *Journal of Religion and Spirituality in Social Work*, *25*(1), 87–106.

Lipka, M., & Majudmar, S. (2019). How religious restrictions around the world have changed over a decade. *Pew Research Center*. Retrieved from https://www.pewresearch.org/fact-tank/2019/07/16/how-religious-restrictions-around-the-world-have-changed-over-a-decade/.

Littman-Ovadia, H., & David, A. (2020). Character strengths as manifestations of spiritual life: Realising the non-dual from the dual. *Frontiers in Psychology*, *11*, 960.

Liu, B. C. C., & Vaughn, M. S. (2019). Legal and policy issues from the U.S. and internationally about mandatory reporting of child abuse. *International Journal of Law and Psychiatry, 64*(May–June), 219–229.

Lloyd, C. E. M., & Kotera, Y. (2021). Mental distress, stigma and help-seeking in the evangelical Christian church: Study protocol. *Journal of Concurrent Disorders*, 1–9.

Loewenthal, K. M., & Lewis, C. A. (2011). Mental health, religion and culture. *The Psychologist, 24*, 256–259.

Lomax, J. W., Karff, S., & McKenny, G. P. (2002). Ethical considerations in the integration of religion and psychotherapy: Three perspectives. *Psychiatric Clinics of North America, 25*, 547–559.

Long, I. J. (2017). Supporting victims of spiritual abuse. *Institute for Muslim Mental Health*. Retrieved from https://muslimmentalhealth.com/supporting-victims-of-spiritual-abuse/.

Lucas-Thompson, R. G., Broderick, P. C., Coatsworth, J. D., & Smyth, J. M. (2019). New avenues for promoting mindfulness in adolescence using mHealth. *Journal of Child and Family Studies, 28*(1), 131–139.

Lüddeckens, D. (2018). Complementary and alternative medicine (CAM) as a toolkit for secular health-care. In D. Lüddekens & M. Schrimp (Eds.), *Medicine — Religion — Spirituality: Global Perspectives on Traditional, Complementary, and Alternative Healing* (pp. 167–200). Transcript Verlag.

Lukoff, D. (1998). From spiritual emergency to spiritual problem: the transpersonal roots of the new DSM-IV category. *Journal of Humanistic Psychology, 38*(2), 21–50.

Lukoff, D. (2007a). Spirituality in the recovery from persistent mental disorders. *Southern Medical Journal, 100*(6), 642–646.

Lukoff, D. (2007b). Visionary spiritual experiences. *Southern Medical Journal, 100*(6), 635–641.

Ma, H. K. (1988). The Chinese perspectives on moral judgment development. *International Journal of Psychology, 23*, 201–227.

Magaldi-Dopman, D., & Park-Taylor, J. (2013). Sacred adolescence: Practical suggestions for psychologists working with adolescents' religious and spiritual identity. *Spirituality in Clinical Practice, 1*(S), 40–52.

Mahoney, A., Flint, D. D., & McGraw, J. S. (2020). Spirituality, religion, and mood disorders. In D. H. Rosmarin & H. G. Koenig (Eds.), *Handbook of Spirituality, Religion, and Mental Health* (pp. 159–177). Elsevier Science and Technology.

Manjapra, K. (2020). *Colonialism in Global Perspective*. Cambridge University Press.

Manning, L. K. (2012). Experiences from Pagan women: A closer look at croning rituals. *Journal of Aging Studies, 26*(1), 102–108.

Marzband, R., Hosseini, S. H., & Hamzehgardeshi, Z. (2016). A concept analysis of spiritual care based on Islamic sources. *Religions, 7*(61), 2–11.

Maslow, A. H. (1943). A theory of human motivation. *Psychological Review, 50*(4), 370–396.

Maslow, A. H. (1964). *Religions, Values, and Peak Experiences.* Penguin Books.

Mattern, S. P. (2016). Galen's anxious patients: Lypē as anxiety disorder. In G. Petridou & C. Thumiger (Eds.), *Homo Patiens: Approaches to the Patient in the Ancient World* (pp. 206–233). Brill.

Mbow, C., *et al.* (2019). Food security. In P. R. Shukla, *et al.* (Eds.), *Climate Change and Land: an IPCC Special Report on Climate Change, Desertification, Land Degradation, Sustainable Land Management, Food Security, and Greenhouse Gas Fluxes in Terrestrial Ecosystems* (pp. 437–550). Intergovernmental Panel on Climate Change.

McCornack, S., & Ortiz, J. (2017). *Choices and Connections: An Introduction to Communication.* St. Martins.

Mcgruder, J. H. (1999). Madness in Zanzibar: Schizophrenia in three families in the Third World. *Dissertation Abstracts International Section A: Humanities and Social Sciences, 60*(4-A), 1208.

McKinlay, E. (2006). *Spiritual Growth and Care in the Fourth Age of Life.* Jessica Kingsley Publishers.

Mead, G. H. (1934). *Mind, Self, and Society.* University of Chicago Press.

Mercer, J. (2014). International concerns about holding therapy. *Research on Social Work Practice, 24*(2), 188–191.

Memaryan, N., Rassouli, M., & Mehrabi, M. (2016). Spirituality concept by health professionals in Iran: A qualitative study. *Evidence-Based Complementary and Alternative Medicine, 2016*, 8913870.

Messias, E., Pesechkian, H., & Cagande, C. (2020). *Positive Psychiatry, Psychotherapy, and Psychology: Clinical Applications.* Springer.

Miller, M. M., *et al.* (2007). Integrating spirituality into training: The spiritual issues in supervision scale. *The American Journal of Family Therapy, 34*(4), 355–372.

Milner, K., Crawford, P., Edgley, A., Hare-Duke, L., & Slade, M. (2020). The experiences of spirituality among adults with mental health difficulties: a qualitative systematic review. *Epidemiology and Psychiatric Sciences, 29*, E34.

Moaddel, M., & Karabenick, S. A. (2018). Religious fundamentalism in eight Muslim-majority countries: Reconceptualization and assessment. *Journal for the Scientific Study of Religion, 57*(4), 676–706.

Moodley, R., & West, W. (2005). *Integrating Traditional Healing Practices into Counseling and Psychotherapy.* SAGE Publications.

Moody, R. A. (1975). *Life after Life.* Bantam.

Mooney, C. G. (2009). *Theories of Attachment: An Introduction to Bowlby, Ainsworth, Gerber, Brazelton, Kennell, and Klause.* Redleaf Press.

Moore, L. E., & Greyson, B. (2017). Characteristics of memories for near-death experiences. *Consciousness and Cognition, 51*, 116–124.

Moreira-Almeida, A., Sharma, A., van Rensberg, B. J., Verhagen, P. J., Cook, C. C. H. (2016). WPA position statement on spirituality and religion in psychiatry. *World Psychiatry, 15*(1), 87–88.

Mosqueiro, B. P., Pinto, A. de R., & Moreira-Almeida, A. (2020). Spirituality, religion, and mood disorders. In D. H. Rosmarin & H. G. Koenig (Eds.), *Handbook of Spirituality, Religion, and Mental Health* (pp. 1–25). Elsevier Science & Technology.

Motlagh, F. E., Ibrahim, F., Rashid, R. A., Seghatoleslam, T., & Habil, H. (2016). Acupuncture therapy for drug addiction. *Chinese Medicine, 11*(16), 1–20.

Mowat, H. (2011). Voicing the spiritual: Working with people with dementia. In A. Jewell (Ed.), *Spirituality and Personhood in Dementia* (pp. 75–86). Jessica Kingsley Publishers.

Mruk, C. J., & Hartzell, J. (2003). *Zen and Psychotherapy: Integrating Traditional and Nontraditional Approaches.* Springer.

Muggah, R., & Velshi, A. (2019). Religious violence is on the rise. What can faith-based communities do about it. *World Economic Forum.* Retrieved from https://www.weforum.org/agenda/2019/02/how-should-faith-communities-halt-the-rise-in-religious-violence/.

Mukherjee, A. (2002). Hindu Psychology and the Bhagavad Gita. In R. Olson (Ed.), *Religious Theories of Personality and Psychotherapy: East Meets West* (pp. 19–84). Routledge.

Murphy, P. E., Fitchett, G., & Emery Tigurcio, E. (2016). Religious and spiritual struggle: Prevalence and correlates among older adults with depression in the BRIGHTEN program. *Mental Health, Religion, and Culture, 19*, 713–721.

NADA (n.d.). Michael Smith. *NADA.* Retrieved from https://acudetox.com/about-nada/michael-smith/.

Naimi, E., Babuei, A., Moslemirad, M., Rezaei, R., & Eilami, O. (2021). The effect of spirituality intervention on the anxiety of parents of hospitalized newborns in a neonatal department. *Journal of Religion and Health, 60*, 354–361.

Naor, L., & Mayseless, O. (2019). The therapeutic value of experiencing spirituality in nature. *Spirituality in Clinical Practice, 7*(2), 114–133.

Narayanaswamy, V. (1981). Origin and development of Ayurveda (A brief history). *Ancient Science of Life, 1*(1), 1–7.

National Association of Social Workers. (2001). Cultural competence in the social work profession. In *Social Work Speaks: NASW Policy Statements* (pp. 59–62). National Association for Social Workers.

National Association of Social Workers. (2020). Social workers must help dismantle systems of oppression and fight racism within social work profession. *National Association of Social Workers.* Retrieved from https://www.socialworkers.org/News/News-Releases/ID/2219/Social-Workers-Must-Help-Dismantle-Systems-of-Oppression-and-Fight-Racism-Within-Social-Work-Profession.

National Association of Social Workers. (2021). National Association of Social Workers Code of Ethics. *National Association of Social Workers.* Retrieved from https://www.socialworkers.org/About/Ethics/Code-of-Ethics/Code-of-Ethics-English.

National Institute for Mental Health. (n.d.). Mental Illness. *National Institute for Mental Health.* Retrieved from https://www.nimh.nih.gov/health/statistics/mental-illness.

National Institutes of Health (2021). Complementary and Alternative Medicine. *National Institute of Health.* Retrieved from https://www.cancer.gov/about-cancer/treatment/cam.

National Working Group on Child Abuse Linked to Faith or Belief. (2012). National action plan to tackle child abuse linked to faith or belief. *Department for Education.* Retrieved from https://www.gov.uk/government/news/action-plan-to-stop-child-abuse-in-the-name-of-faith-or-belief.

Nelson, J. M. (2009). *Psychology, Religion, and Spirituality.* Springer.

Nelson, C. A., Fox, N. A., & Zeanah, C. (2013). Anguish of the abandoned child. *Scientific American, 308*(4), 62–67.

Newberg, A. (2021). *Neurotheology: How Science Can Enlighten Us About Spirituality.* Columbia University Press.

Nguyen, H. (2018). Exploring perceptions of mental health clients and professionals about Buddhism-based therapies at mental health hospitals in Vietnam. *Asian Social Work and Policy Review*, 12(2), 94–107.

Niemiec, R. M., Fusso-Netzer, P., & Pargament, K. I. (2020). The decoding of the human spirituality: A synergy of spiritual and character strengths toward wholeness. *Frontiers in Psychology, 11*, 2040.

Nieuwsma, J., Walser, R., Hayes, S., & Tan, S. (2016). *ACT for Clergy and Pastoral Counselors: Using Acceptance and Commitment Therapy to Bridge Psychological and Spiritual Care.* Context Press.

Nolan, P., & Lenski, G. (2014). *Human Societies: An Introduction to Macrosociology* (12th ed.). Oxford University Press.

Norman, S. B., & Maguen, S. (n.d.). Moral Injury. *U.S. Department of Veterans Affairs*. Retrieved from https://www.ptsd.va.gov/professional/treat/cooccurring/moral_injury.asp.

Nye, M. (2018). On how the category of religion is a part of settler colonial power. *Religion Bites (Blog)*. Retrieved from https://medium.com/religion-bites/on-how-the-category-of-religion-is-a-part-of-settler-colonial-power-a9d5db-de3ca3.

Oakley, L., & Kinmond, K. (2013). Introduction. In L. Oakley & K. Kinmond (Eds.), *Breaking the Silence on Spiritual Abuse* (p. 151). Palgrave Macmillan.

Oliver, P. (2012). *New Religious Movements: A Guide for the Perplexed*. Continuum.

Olson, R. P. (2002). *Religious Theories of Personality and Psychotherapy: East Meets West*. Routledge.

Oman, D. (2018). *Why Religion and Spirituality Matter for Public Health*. Springer.

O'Neill, K. (2020). Integrating expressive arts therapy and spirituality: A literature review of trauma treatment. *Expressive Therapies Capstone Thesis*. Retrieved from https://digitalcommons.lesley.edu/cgi/viewcontent.cgi?article=1373&context=expressive_theses.

Owen, J. (2005). Farming claims almost half Earth's land, new maps show. *National Geographic*. Retrieved from https://www.nationalgeographic.com/history/article/agriculture-food-crops-land#:~:text=New%20maps%20show%20food%20production,of%20the%20planet%2C%20scientists%20say.&text=Food%20production%20takes%20up%20almost,that%20still%20remains%2C%20scientists%20warn.

Oxhandler, H. K., Parrish, D. E., Torres, L. R., & Achenbum, W. A. (2015). The integration of clients' religion and spirituality in social work practice: A national survey. *Social Work*, *60*(3), 228–237.

Oxhandler, H. K., & Parrish, D. E. (2017). Integrating clients' religion/spirituality in clinical practice: A comparison among social workers, psychologists, counselors, marriage and family therapists, and nurses. *Journal of Clinical Psychology*, *64*(4), 680–694.

Oxhandler, H. K., Polson, E. C., & Achenbaum, W. A. (2018). The religiosity and spiritual beliefs and practices of clinical social workers: A national survey. *Social Work*, *63*(1), 47–56.

Pandya, S. P. (2018a). Spirituality for mental health and well-being of adult refugees in Europe. *Journal of Immigrant and Minority Health*, *20*(6), 1396–1404.

Pandya, S. P. (2018b). Spiritual counseling program for children with anxiety disorders: A multi-city experiment. *Journal of Pastoral Care and Counseling*, *72*(1), 45–57.

Pargament, K. I., & Brant, C. R. (1998). Religion and coping. In D. H. Rosmarin & H. G. Koenig (Eds.), *Handbook of Religion and Mental Health* (pp. 112–129). Academic Press.

Pargament, K. I., & Saunders, S. M. (2007). Introduction to the special issue on spirituality and psychotherapy. *Journal of Clinical Psychology, 63*(10), 903–907.

Pargament, K. I. (2013). *APA Handbook of Psychology, Religion, and Spirituality.* American Psychological Association (APA).

Pargament, K. I., & Lomax, J. W. (2013). Understanding and addressing religion among people with mental illness. *World Psychiatry, 12*(1), 26–32.

Pargament, K. I., & Exline, J. J. (2020). Religious and spiritual struggles. *American Psychological Association.* Retrieved from https://www.apa.org/research/action/religious-spiritual-struggles.

Park, C. L., Currier, J. M., Harris, I., & Slattery, J. M. (2017). *Trauma, Meaning, and Spirituality: Research into Clinical Practice.* American Psychological Association.

Pearce, M. J., *et al.* (2015). Religiously integrated cognitive behavioral therapy: A new method of treatment for major depression in patients with chronic mental illness. *Psychotherapy, 52*(1), 56–66.

Pearson, J. (2002). *Belief Beyond Boundaries: Wicca, Celtic Spirituality, and the New Age.* Ashgate Press.

Pendergast, S., & Pendergast, T. (2000). *St. James Encyclopedia of Popular Culture.* St. James Press.

Penelope, J. (2019). Six reasons to stop using the word shaman. *Patheos.* Retrieved from https://www.patheos.com/blogs/thewanderingwitch/2019/03/6-reasons-you-should-stop-using-the-word-shaman/.

Pesut, B. (2008). A conversation on diverse perspectives of spirituality in nursing home literature. *Nursing Philosophy, 9*, 98–109.

Pesut, B., Fowler, M., Taylor, E. J., Reimer-Kirkham, S., & Sawatzky, R. (2008). Conceptualising spirituality and religion for healthcare. *Journal of Clinical Nursing, 17*(21), 2803–2810.

Peteet, J. R. (2014). What is the place of clinicians' religious or spiritual commitments in psychotherapy? A virtues-based perspective. *Journal of Religion and Health, 53*, 1190–1198.

Peteet, J. R. (2019). Approaching religiously reinforced mental health stigma: A conceptual framework. *Psychiatric Services, 70*(9), 846–848.

Peterson, C., & Seligman, M. E. P. (2004). *Character Strengths and Virtues: A Handbook and Classification.* Oxford University Press and American Psychological Association.

Peterson, C. (2008). What is positive psychology and what is it not? *Psychology Today*. Retrieved from https://www.psychologytoday.com/us/blog/the-good-life/200805/what-is-positive-psychology-and-what-is-it-not.

Petkari, E., & Ortiz-Tallo, M. (2018). Towards youth happiness and mental health in the United Arab Emirates: The path of character strengths in a multicultural population. *Journal of Happiness Studies*, *19*, 333–350.

Pew Forum on Religion and Public Life. (2009). Faith in flux. *Pew Research Center*. Retrieved from http://www.pewforum.org/2009/04/27/faith-in-flux.

Pew Research Center. (2012). The global religious landscape. *Pew Research Center*. Retrieved from https://www.pewforum.org/2012/12/18/global-religious-landscape-exec/.

Pew Research Center. (2017a). More Americans now say they're spiritual but not religious. *Pew Research Center*. Retrieved from https://www.pewresearch.org/fact-tank/2017/09/06/more-americans-now-say-theyre-spiritual-but-not-religious/.

Pew Research Center. (2017b). U.S. Muslims concerned about their place in society, but continue to believe in the American dream. *Pew Research Center*. Retrieved from https://www.pewforum.org/2017/07/26/religious-beliefs-and-practices/.

Pew Research Center. (2018). Being Christian in western Europe. *Pew Research Center*. Retrieved from https://www.pewforum.org/2018/05/29/attitudes-toward-spirituality-and-religion/.

Pew Research Center. (2019). 10 facts about atheists. *Pew Research Center*. Retrieved from https://www.pewresearch.org/fact-tank/2019/12/06/10-facts-about-atheists/.

Pew Research Center. (2020a). The global god divide. *Pew Research Center*. Retrieved from https://www.pewresearch.org/global/2020/07/20/the-global-god-divide/.

Pew Research Center. (2020b). In 2018, Government restrictions on religion reach highest level globally in more than a decade. *Pew Research Center*. Retrieved from https://www.pewforum.org/2020/11/10/in-2018-government-restrictions-on-religion-reach-highest-level-globally-in-more-than-a-decade/.

Pfeifer, S. (2007). Biblical themes in psychiatric practice. In G. Glas, M. H. Spero, P. J. Verhagen, & H. M. van Pragg (Eds.), *Hearing Visions, Seeing Voices* (pp. 267–277). Springer.

Pharo, L. K. (2011). A methodology for a deconstruction and reconstruction of the concepts "shaman" and "shamanism". *Numan*, *58*, 6–70.

Piaget, J. (1977). *The Essential Piaget*. Basic Books.

Pies, R. W., & Geppert, C. (2013). Ethical issues in the psychiatric treatment of the religious "fundamentalist" patient. *Medscape*. Retrieved from https://www.

psychologists.bc.ca/sites/default/files/pdfs/other_pdfs/Ethical%20Issues%20
Treating%20Religious%20Fundamentalist%20Patient.pdf.

Plante, T. G. (2007). Integrating spirituality and psychotherapy: Ethical issues and principles to consider. *Journal of Clinical Psychology, 63*, 891–902.

Plante, T. G. (2009). *Spiritual Practices in Psychotherapy: Thirteen Tools for Enhancing Psychological Health.* American Psychological Association.

Pollan, M. (2019). *How to Change Your Mind: What the New Science of Psychedelics Teaches Us About Consciousness, Dying, Addiction, Depression, and Transcendence.* Penguin Press.

Porges, S. W. (2011). *The Polyvagal Theory.* W.W. Norton.

Porges, S. W. (2019). Dr. Stephen Porges speaks about spirituality concepts from a polyvagal perspective. *Integrated Listening Systems.* Retrieved from https://integratedlistening.com/dr-stephen-porges-speaks-about-spirituality-concepts-from-a-polyvagal-perspective/.

Pratt, D. (2010). Religion and terrorism: Christian fundamentalism and extremism. *Terrorism and Political Violence, 22*(3), 438–456.

Prieto-Ursúa, M., & Jódar, R. (2020). Finding meaning in hell. The role of meaning, religiosity and spirituality in posttraumatic growth during the coronavirus crisis in Spain. *Frontiers in Psychology, 11*, 567836.

Progoff, I. (1973). *Jung's Psychology and its Social Meaning.* Anchor Books.

Pryce, J., & Walsh, F. (2003). The spiritual dimension of family life. In F. Walsh (Ed.), *Normal Family Processes: Growing Diversity and Complexity* (pp. 337–375). Guilford Press.

Pulchaski, C. (2006). Spiritual assessment in clinical practice. *Psychiatric Annals, 36*(3), 150–155.

Qureshi, N. A., Khalil, A. A., & Alsanad, S. M. (2018). Spiritual and religious healing practices: Some reflections from Saudi National Center for complementary and alternative medicine, Riyadh. *Journal of Religion and Health, 59*, 845–869.

Rabinowitz, A. (2010). *Judaic Spiritual Psychotherapy.* University Press of America.

Ragins, M. (2006). *Recovery with Severe Mental Illness: Changing from A Medical Model to a Psychosocial Rehabilitation Model.* National Mental Health Consumers' Self-Help Clearinghouse.

Rajpal, S. (2020). *Curing Madness? A Social and Cultural History of Insanity in Colonial North India, 1800–1950s.* Oxford University Press.

Rambo, L. R. (1993). *Understanding Religious Conversion.* Yale University Press.

Rangaswami, K. (1992). Indian model of stages in human development and developmental tasks. *Indian Journal of Psychological Medicine, 15*, 77–82.

Rasmussen, S. J. (2000). From childbearers to culture-bearers: Transition to postchildbearing among Tuareg women. *Medical Anthropology, 19*, 91–116.

Rayes, D., Karnouk, C., Churbaji, D., Walther, L., & Bajbouj, M. (2021). Faith-based coping among arabic-speaking refugees seeking mental health services in Berlin, Germany: An exploratory qualitative study. *Frontiers in Psychology*, *12*, 595979.

Redfield, R. (1947). The folk society. *American Journal of Sociology*, *52*(4), 293–308.

Reid, K. (2021). Forced to flee: Top countries refugees are coming from. *World Vision*. Retrieved from https://www.worldvision.org/refugees-news-stories/forced-to-flee-top-countries-refugees-coming-from.

Reiff, C. M., *et al.* (2020). Psychedelics and psychedelic-assisted therapy. *American Journal of Psychiatry*, *177*(5), 391–410.

Reinert, K. G., *et al.* (2016). The role of religious involvement in the relationship between early trauma and health outcomes among adult survivors. *Journal of Child and Adolescent Trauma, 9*, 231–241.

Reynolds, D. K. (1976). *Morita Psychotherapy*. University of California Press.

Richards, P. S., & Worthington, E. L. Jr. (2010). The need for evidence-based, spiritually oriented psychotherapies. *Professional Psychology: Research and Practice*, *41*, 363–370.

Richards, P. S., & Bergin, A. E. (2014). *Handbook of Psychotherapy and Religious Diversity* (2nd ed.). American Psychological Association.

Richards, P. S., Sanders, P. W., Lea, T., McBride, J. A., & Allen, G. (2015). Bringing spiritually oriented psychotherapies into the health care mainstream: A call for worldwide collaboration. *Spirituality in Clinical Practice*, *2*(3), 169–179.

Richards, P. S., Weinberger-Litman, S., Berrett, M. E., & Hardman, R. K. (2020). In D. H. Rosmarin & H. G. Koenig (Eds.), *Handbook of Spirituality, Religion, and Mental Health* (pp. 99–118). Elsevier Science & Technology.

Rickhi, B., Kania-Richmond, A., Moritz, S., Cohen, J., Paccagnan, P., Dennis, C., Liu, M., Malhotra, S., Steele, P., & Toews, J. (2015). Evaluation of a spirituality informed e-mental health tool as an intervention for major depressive disorder in adolescents and young adults — a randomized controlled pilot trial. *BMX Complementary and Alternative Medicine*, *15*, 450.

Rider, C. (2011). Medical magic and the church in thirteenth-century England. *Social History of Medicine*, *24*(1), 92–107.

Rogers, C. (1951). *Client-Centered Therapy: Its Current Practice, Implications, and Theory*. Houghton Mifflin.

Ronald, R., & Alexy, A. (2011). *Home and Family in Japan: Continuity and Transformation*. Routledge.

Roseneil, S., Crowhurst, I., Hellesund, T., Santos, A. C., & Stoilova, M. (2020). *The Tenacity of the Couple Norm: Intimate Citizenship Regimes in a Changing Europe*. University College London Press.

Rosmarin, D. H., Malloy, M. C., & Forester, B. P. (2014). Spiritual struggle and affective symptoms among geriatric mood disordered patients. *International Journal of Geriatric Psychiatry*, *29*, 653–660.

Rosmarin, D. H., & Koenig, H. G. (2020). Introduction. In D. H. Rosmarin & H. G. Koenig (Eds.), *Handbook of Spirituality, Religion, and Mental Health* (pp. xvii–xxiv). Elsevier Science and Technology.

Rosmarin, D. H., & Leidl, B. (2020). Spirituality, religion, and anxiety disorders. In D. H. Rosmarin & H. G. Koenig (Eds.), *Handbook of Spirituality, Religion, and Mental Health* (pp. 41–60). Elsevier Science & Technology.

Ross, D. K., Suprina, J. S., & Brack, G. (2013). The spirituality in supervision model (SACRED): An emerging model from a meta-synthesis of the literature. *The Practitioner Scholar: Journal of Counseling and Professional Psychology*, *2*, 68–83.

Roszak, T. (1992). *The Voice of the Earth*. Simon & Schuster.

Roszak, T., & Gomes, M. (1995). *Ecopsychology: Restoring the Earth, Healing the Mind*. Counterpoint.

Rouholamini, M., Kalantarkousheh, S. M., & Sharifi, E. (2017). Effectiveness of spiritual components training on life satisfaction of Persian orphan adolescents. *Journal of Religion and Health*, *56*(6), 1895–1902.

Rouse, L. (2014). American Indian traditional ways: Convergence and divergence with positive psychology. In C. Kim-Prieto (Ed.), *Religion and Spirituality across Cultures* (pp. 137–161). Springer.

Rubenstein, R. L., Girling, L. M., de Medeiros, K., & Brazda, M. (2015). Expanding the framework of generativity theory through research: A qualitative study. *The Gerontologist*, *55*(4), 548–559.

Rust, M-J. (2020). *Towards an Ecopschotherapy*. Confer Books.

Saad, M., de Medeiros, R., & Mosini, A. C. (2017). Are we ready for a true biopsychosocial-spiritual model? The many meanings of "spiritual". *Medicines*, *4*(4), 79.

Saguil, A., & Phelps, K. (2012). The spiritual assessment. *American Family Physician*, *86*(6), 546–550.

Saitō, T. (2012). *Social Withdrawal: Adolescence without End*. University of Minnesota Press.

Sangree, W. H. (1987). The childless elderly in Tiriki, Kenya, and Irigwe, Nigeria: A comparative analysis of the relationship between beliefs about childlessness and the social status of the childless elderly. *Journal of Cross-Cultural Gerontology*, *2*, 201–223.

Saunders, S. M., Miller, M. L., & Bright, M. M. (2010). Spiritually conscious psychological care. *Professional Psychology: Research and Practice*, *41*(5), 355–362.

Sayadmansour, A. (2014). Neurotheology: The relationship between brain and religion. *Iranian Journal of Neurology*, *13*(1), 52–55.

Schiffman, R. (2019). When religion leads to trauma. *The New York Times*. Retrieved from https://www.nytimes.com/2019/02/05/well/mind/religion-trauma-lgbt-gay-depression-anxiety.html.

Schleutker, E. (2020). Co-optation and repression of religion in authoritarian regimes. *Politics and Religion*, *14*(2), 1–32.

Schroeder, S. (n.d.) Mental illness and families of faith: How congregations can respond. *Mental Health Ministries*. Retrieved from https://www.naminh.org/wp-content/uploads/2017/08/MHM-MI-StudyGuide.pdf.

Schultz, C., Walker, R., Bessarab, D., McMillan, F., McLeod, J., & Marriatt, R. (2014). Interdisciplinary care to enhance mental health and social and emotional wellbeing. In P. Dudgeon, H. Milroy, & R. Parker (Eds.), *Working Together: Aboriginal and Torres Strait Islander Mental Health and Wellbeing Principles and Practice* (pp. 221–242). Australian Government, Telethon Institute for Child Health Research/Kulunga Research Network, and University of Western Australia.

Scull, A. (2015). *Madness in Civilization*. Princeton University Press.

Seligman, M. E. P., & Csikszentmihalyi, M. (2000). Special issue on happiness, excellence, and optimal human functioning. *American Psychologist*, *55*(5), 5–183.

Seligman, M. E. P. (2011). *Flourish: A Visionary New Understanding of Happiness and Well-being*. Free Press.

Senchuk, D. M. (1990). Listening to a different voice: A feminist critique of Gilligan. *Studies in Philosophy and Education*, *10*, 233–249.

Senreich, E. (2013). An inclusive definition of spirituality for social work education and practice. *Journal of Social Work Education*, *49*(4), 548–563.

Shafranske, E. P. (2014). Addressing religiousness and spirituality as clinically relevant cultural features in supervision. In C. A. Falender, E. P. Shafranske, & C. J. Falicov (Eds.), *Multiculturalism and Diversity in Clinical Supervision: A Competency-Based Approach* (pp. 181–207). American Psychological Association.

Shupe, A. (2007). *No Spoils of the Kingdom: Clergy Misconduct and Religious Community*. University of Illinois Press.

Simon, E. (2020). What Viktor Frankl's logotherapy can offer in the Anthropocene. *Aeon*. Retrieved from https://aeon.co/ideas/what-viktor-frankls-logotherapy-can-offer-in-the-anthropocene.

Simonic, B., Mandell, T. R., & Novsak, R. (2013). Religious-related abuse in the family. *Journal of Family Violence*, *28*(4), 339–349.

Sinha, V. (2007). Folk Hinduism. In *The Blackwell Encyclopedia of Sociology* (ebook). John Wiley & Sons.

Smith, W. C. (1991). *The Meaning and End of Religion*. Fortress Press.

Sokolove, D. (2021). Meeting the Divine. Online class. Seekers Church, Washington, DC.

South, S. J., & Lei, L. (2015). Failures-to-launch and boomerang kids: Contemporary determinants of leaving and returning to the parental home. *Social Forces, 94*(2), 863–890.

St. Arnaud, K., & Cormier, D. (2017). Psychosis or spiritual emergency: The potential of developmental psychopathology for differential diagnosis. *International Journal of Transpersonal Studies, 36*(2), 44–59.

Stanford, M. S., & McAlister, K. R. (2008). Perceptions of serious mental illness in the local church. *Journal of Religion Disability & Health, 12*(2), 144–153.

Stanley, M. A., Bush, A. L., Camp, M. E., Jameson, J. P., Philips, L. L., Barber, C. R., & Cully, J. A. (2011). Older adults' preferences for religion/spirituality in treatment for anxiety and depression. *Aging and Mental Health, 15*, 334–343.

Stark, R. (2008). *What Americans Really Believe.* Baylor University Press.

Starr, K. (2017). Scars of the soul: Get refusal and spiritual abuse in Orthodox Jewish communities. *Journal of Jewish Women's Studies & Gender, 31*, 37–60.

Stetka, B. (2017). Extended adolescence: When 25 is the new 18. *Scientific American.* Retrieved from https://www.scientificamerican.com/article/extended-adolescence-when-25-is-the-new-181/.

Struthers, R., Eschiti, V. S., & Patchell, B. (2004). Traditional indigenous healing: Part I. *Complementary Therapies in Nursing & Midwifery, 10*, 141–149.

Substance Abuse and Mental Health Services Administration. (2019). *Behavioral Health Services for American Indians and Alaska Natives.* Substance Abuse and Mental Health Services Administration.

Substance Abuse and Mental Health Services Administration. (n.d.). LEARN THE EIGHT DIMENSIONS OF WELLNESS. *Substance Abuse and Mental Health Services Administration.* Retrieved from https://store.samhsa.gov/sites/default/files/d7/priv/sma16-4953.pdf.

Sumaktoyo, N. (2018). Measuring religious intolerance across Indonesian provinces. *New Mandala.* Retrieved from https://www.newmandala.org/measuring-religious-intolerance-across-indonesian-provinces/.

Summers, J. K., & Vivian, D. N. (2018). Ecotherapy — a forgotten ecosystem service: A review. *Frontiers in Psychotherapy, 9*, 1389.

Tajan, N., Hamasaki, Y., & Pionnié-Dax, N. (2017). Hikikomori: The Japanese Cabinet Office's 2016 survey of acute social withdrawal. *The Asia-Pacific Journal: Japan Focus, 15*(5), 5017.

Taku, K., & McDiarmid, L. (2015) Personally important posttraumatic growth in adolescents: The effect on self-esteem beyond commonly defined posttraumatic growth. *Journal of Adolescence, 44*, 224–231.

Tasca, C., Rapetti, M., Carta, M. G., & Fadda, B. (2012). Women and hysteria in the history of mental health. *Clinical Practice & Epidemiology in Mental Health, 8*, 110–119.

Taylor, K. E. (2012). *The Brain Supremacy*. Oxford University Press.

Taylor, S. (2016). Breakdowns and 'Shift-Ups'. *Psychology Today*. Retrieved from https://www.psychologytoday.com/us/blog/out-the-darkness/201602/breakdowns-and-shift-ups.

Tedeschi, R. G., & Calhoun, L. G. (2004). *Posttraumatic Growth: Conceptual Foundation and Empirical Evidence*. Lawrence Erlbaum Associates.

Tedeschi, R. G. (2020). Growth after trauma. *Harvard Business Review*. Retrieved from https://hbr.org/2020/07/growth-after-trauma.

Tedlock, B. (2005). *The Woman in the Shaman's Body*. Bantam.

Tervalon, M., & Murray-Garcia, J. (1998). Cultural humility versus cultural competence: A critical distinction in defining physician training outcomes in multicultural education. *Journal of Health Care for the Poor and Underserved, 9*, 117–125.

Thielman, S. (1998). Reflections on the role of religion in the history of psychiatry. In D. H. Rosmarin & H. G. Koenig (Eds.), *Handbook of Religion and Mental Health* (pp. 3–20). Academic Press.

Thorne, B. (2002). *The Mystical Power of Person-Centered Therapy*. John Wiley & Sons.

Tillich, P. (2011). *Dynamics of Faith*. HarperOne.

Tornstam, L. (1989). Gero-transcendence: a meta-theoretical formulation of the disengagement theory. *Aging: Clinical and Experimental Research, 1*(1), 318–326.

Tornstam, L. (2005). *Gerotranscendence: A Developmental Theory of Positive Aging*. Springer.

UNICEF. (2010). From commitment to action: What religious communities can do to eliminate violence against children. *UNICEF.* Retrieved from https://www.unicef.org/media/files/What_Religious_Communities_can_do_to_Eliminate_Violence_against_Children__(UNICEF_Religions_for_Peace_Guide).pdf.

UNICEF. (2020). Child marriage around the world. *UNICEF.* Retrieved from https://www.unicef.org/protection/child-marriage.

United Nations. (1948). Universal Declaration of Human Rights, G.A. res. 217A (III), U.N. Doc A/810 at 71 (1948/1998). *United Nations.* Retrieved from https://www.un.org/en/about-us/universal-declaration-of-human-rights.

United Nations Human Rights Council. (2011). Combatting intolerance, negative stereotyping and stigmatization of, and discrimination, incitement to violence and violence against, persons based on religious belief. *United Nations.*

Retrieved   from   https://www2.ohchr.org/english/bodies/hrcouncil/docs/16session/A.HRC.RES.16.18_en.pdf.

United Nations Population Division. (2016). Changing patterns of marriage and unions across the world. *United Nations.* Retrieved from https://www.un.org/development/desa/pd/sites/www.un.org.development.desa.pd/files/files/documents/2020/Jan/un_2016_factsheet2.pdf.

Unterrainer, H. F., Ruttinger, J., Lewis, A. J., Anglim, J., Fink, A., & Kapfhammer, H. P. (2016). Vulnerable dark triad facets are associated with religious fundamentalist tendencies. *Psychopathology*, *49*, 47–52.

U.S. Census. (2021). Census Bureau Releases New Estimates on America's Families and Living Arrangements. *U.S. Census.* Retrieved from https://www.census.gov/newsroom/press-releases/2021/families-and-living-arrangements.html#:~:text=The%20estimated%20median%20age%20to,stay%2Dat%2Dhome%20father.

U.S. Department of Health and Human Services. (n.d.). HIPAA Privacy Rule and Sharing Information Related to Mental Health. *U.S. Department of Health and Human Services.* Retrieved from https://www.hhs.gov/sites/default/files/hipaa-privacy-rule-and-sharing-info-related-to-mental-health.pdf.

Vaingankar, J. A., Choudhary, N., Chong, S. A., Kumar, F. D. S., & Abdin, E. (2021). Religious affiliation in relation to positive mental health and mental disorders in a multi-ethnic Asian population. *International Journal of Environmental Research and Public Health*, *18*(7), 3368.

Vandenberghe, L., Padro, G. C., & de Camargo, E. A. (2021). Spirituality and religion in psychotherapy: Views of Brazilian psychotherapists. *International Perspectives in Psychology,* 1(2), 79–93.

van den Enden, T., Boom, J., Brugman, D., & Thoma, S. (2019). Stages of moral judgment development: Applying item response theory to Defining Issues Test data. *Journal of Moral Education*, *48*(4), 423–438.

van der Kolk, B. A. (2009). Developmental trauma disorder: towards a rational diagnosis for chronically traumatized children. *Praxis Der Kinderpsychologie Und Kinderpsychiatrie*, *58*(8), 572–586.

Van de Vondervoort, J., & Hamlin, J. K. (2016). Evidence for intuitive morality: Preverbal infants make sociomoral evaluations. *Child Development Perspectives*, *10*(3), 143–148.

van Gennep, A. (1960). *The Rites of Passage.* University of Chicago Press.

Van Lente, E., & Hogan, M. (2020). Understanding the nature of oneness experience in meditators using collective intelligence methods. *Frontiers in Psychology*, *11*, 2092.

Van Rensburg, A. B. R., Poggenpoel, M., Szabo, C. P., & Myburgh, C. P. H. (2014). Referral and collaboration between South African psychiatrists and religious or spiritual advisors: Views from some psychiatrists. *South African Journal of Psychiatry*, *20*(2), 40–45.

Verghese, A. (2008). Spirituality and mental health. *Indian Journal of Psychiatry*, *50*(4), 233–237.

Vermeer, P. (2014). Religion and family life: An overview of current research and suggestions for future research. *Religions*, *5*(2), 402–421.

Victor, S. E., Devendorf, A., Lewis, S., Rottenberg, J., Muehlenkamp, J. J., Stage, D., & Miller, R. (2021). Only human: Mental health difficulties among clinical, counseling, and school psychology faculty and trainees. *Psyarvix*. https://doi.org/10.31234/osf.io/xbfr6.

Vieten, C., Scammell, S., Pilato, R., Ammondson, I., Pargament, K., & Lukoff, D. (2013). Spiritual and religious competencies for psychologists. *Psychology of Religion and Spirituality*, *5*(3), 129–144.

Vieten, C., & Scammell, S. (2015). *Spiritual and Religious Competencies in Clinical Practice*. New Harbinger.

Viorst, J. (1998). *Necessary Losses*. Fireside Books.

Vonk, R., & Visser, A. (2021). An exploration of spiritual superiority: the paradox of self-enhancement. *European Journal of Social Psychology*, *51*, 152–165.

Wadensten, B. (2007). The theory of gerotranscendence as applied to gerontological nursing — Part I. *International Journal of Older Person Nursing*, *2*(4), 289–294.

Walker, L. J. (2003). Morality, religion, spirituality — the value of saintliness. *Journal of Moral Education*, *32*(4), 373–384.

Walker, M. T. (2006). The social construction of mental illness and its implications for the recovery model. *International Journal of Psychosocial Rehabilitations*, *10*(1), 71–87.

Walsh, R., & Vaughan, F. (1993). On transpersonal definitions. *Journal of Transpersonal Psychology*, *25*(2), 125–182.

Warlick, C. A., Lawrence, R., & Armstrong, A. (2021). Examining fundamentalism and mental health in a religiously diverse LGBTQ+ sample. *Spirituality in Clinical Practice*, *8*(2), 149–160.

Watters, E. (2010). *No Crazy Like Us: The Globalization of the American Psyche*. Free Press.

Wellwood, J. (2000). *Toward a Psychology of Awakening*. Shambala Publications.

White, E. D. (2016). *Wicca: History, Belief, and Community in Modern Pagan Witchcraft*. Sussex Academic Press.

Whitley, R., & Jarvis, E. (2015). Religious understanding as cultural competence: Issues for clinicians. *Psychiatric Times*. Retrieved from https://www. psychiatrictimes.com/view/religious-understanding-cultural-competence-issues-clinicians.

Wibisono, S., Louis, W. R., & Jetten, J. (2019). A multidimensional analysis of religious extremism. *Frontiers in Psychology*, *10*, 2560.

Wilber, K. (n.d.). From the great chain of being to postmodernism in three easy steps. *Self-published*. Retrieved from http://www.kenwilber.com/Writings/PDF/FromGC2PM_GENERAL_2005_NN.pdf.

Wilkinson, A. (2018). I didn't read Harry Potter when I was growing up. And I wasn't alone. *Vox*. Retrieved from https://www.vox.com/culture/2018/8/31/17607988/harry-potter-boycott-evangelical-dobson-focus-peretti-satanic-panic.

Wilson, B. (1939). *Alcoholics Anonymous*. TarcherPerigee.

Wilt, J. A., Grubb, J. B., Exline, J. J., & Pargament, K. I. (2016). Personality, religious and spiritual struggles, and well-being. *Psychology of Religion and Spirituality*, *8*(4), 341–351.

Winell, M, (2006). *Leaving the Fold: A Guide for Former Fundamentalists and Others Leaving Their Religion*. Apocryphile Press.

Wink, P., Dillon, M., & Fay, K. (2005). Spiritual seeking, narcissism, and psychotherapy: How are they related? *Journal for the Scientific Study of Religion*, *44*(2), 143–158.

Winkelman, M. J. (1986). Magico-religious practitioner types and socioeconomic analysis. *Behavior Science Research*, *20*, 1–4.

Winslow, G. R., & Wehtje-Winslow, B. J. (2007). Ethical boundaries of spiritual care. *Medical Journal of Australia*, *186*(S10), S63–S66.

Winsor, M. (2018). Why adults in different parts of the globe live at home with their parents. *ABC News*. Retrieved from https://abcnews.go.com/International/adults-parts-globe-live-home-parents/story?id=55457188.

Wong, E. C., Fulton, B. R., & Derose, K. P. (2017). Prevalence and predictors of mental health programming among U.S. religious congregations. *Psychiatric Services*, *69*(2), 154–160.

World Health Organization. (2018). Mental health: strengthening our response. *World Health Organization*. Retrieved from https://www.who.int/news-room/fact-sheets/detail/mental-health-strengthening-our-response.

World Values Survey Association (2014). *Wave 6 2010–2014 OFFICIAL AGGREGATE v.20150418*. World Values Survey Association.

WPA Standing Committee on Ethics and Review. (2020). Code of Ethics for Psychiatry. *World Psychiatric Association*. Retrieved from

https://3ba346de-fde6-473f-b1da-536498661f9c.filesusr.com/ugd/e172f3_4
cecd522c2d448c7944342ba88c527e5.pdf.

Xu, Y. (2020). Professionalism and sustainability of faith-based social work organisations in China. *China: An International Journal, 18*(4), 123–140.

Yamada, A. M., Lukoff, D., Lim, C., & Mancuso, L. L. (2020). Integrating spirituality and mental health: Perspectives of adults receiving public mental health services in California. *Psychology of Religion and Spirituality, 12*(3), 276–287.

Yang, K. S., & Wen, C. I. (1982). *The Sinicization of Social and Behavioral Science Research in China* [in Chinese]. Taipei Institute of Ethnology, Academia Sinica.

Yang, K. S. (1997). Theories and research in Chinese personality: An indigenous approach. In H. S. R. Kao & D. Sinha (Eds.), *Asian Perspectives on Psychology* (pp. 236–262). SAGE Publications.

Yang, W., Staps, T., & Hijmans, E. (2010). Existential crisis and the awareness of dying: The role of meaning and spirituality. *Omega, 61*(1), 53–69.

Yoo, T. J. (2016). *The Politics of Mental Health in Colonial Korea.* University of California Press.

Yoshioka, K. (2020). The '8050 issue' of social withdrawal and poverty in Japan's super-aged society. *Journal of Advanced Nursing, 76*(8), 1884–1885.

Young, M. J., & Sarin, R. (2014). Fostering meaning, social connection, and well-being through Hindu beliefs and practices. In C. Kim-Prieto (Ed.), *Religion and Spirituality across Cultures* (pp. 87–100). Springer.

Yusuf, A. A., Shidiq, A. R., & Hariyadi, H. (2020). On socio-economic predictors of religious intolerance: Evidence from a large-scale longitudinal survey in the largest Muslim democracy. *Religions, 11*(1), 21.

Zare, A., Bahia, N. J., Elidy, F., Adib, N., & Sedighe, F. (2019). The relationship between spiritual well-being, mental health, and quality of life in cancer patients receiving chemotherapy. *Journal of Family Medicine and Primary Care, 8*(5), 1700–1705.

Zhong, W., Cristofori, I., Bulbulia, J., Krueger, F., & Grafman, J. (2017). Biological and cognitive underpinnings of religious fundamentalism. *Neuropsychologia, 100*, 18–25.

Zimmer, A., Jagger, C., Chiu, C-T., Ofstedal, M. B., Rojo, F., & Saito, Y. (2016). Spirituality, religiosity, aging and health in global perspective: A review. *SSM Population Health, 2*, 373–381.

Zimmerman, M., Morgan, T. A., & Stanton, K. (2018). The severity of psychiatric disorders. *World Psychiatry, 17*(3), 258–275.

Zukav, G. (1989). *The Seat of the Soul.* Simon & Schuster.

Index

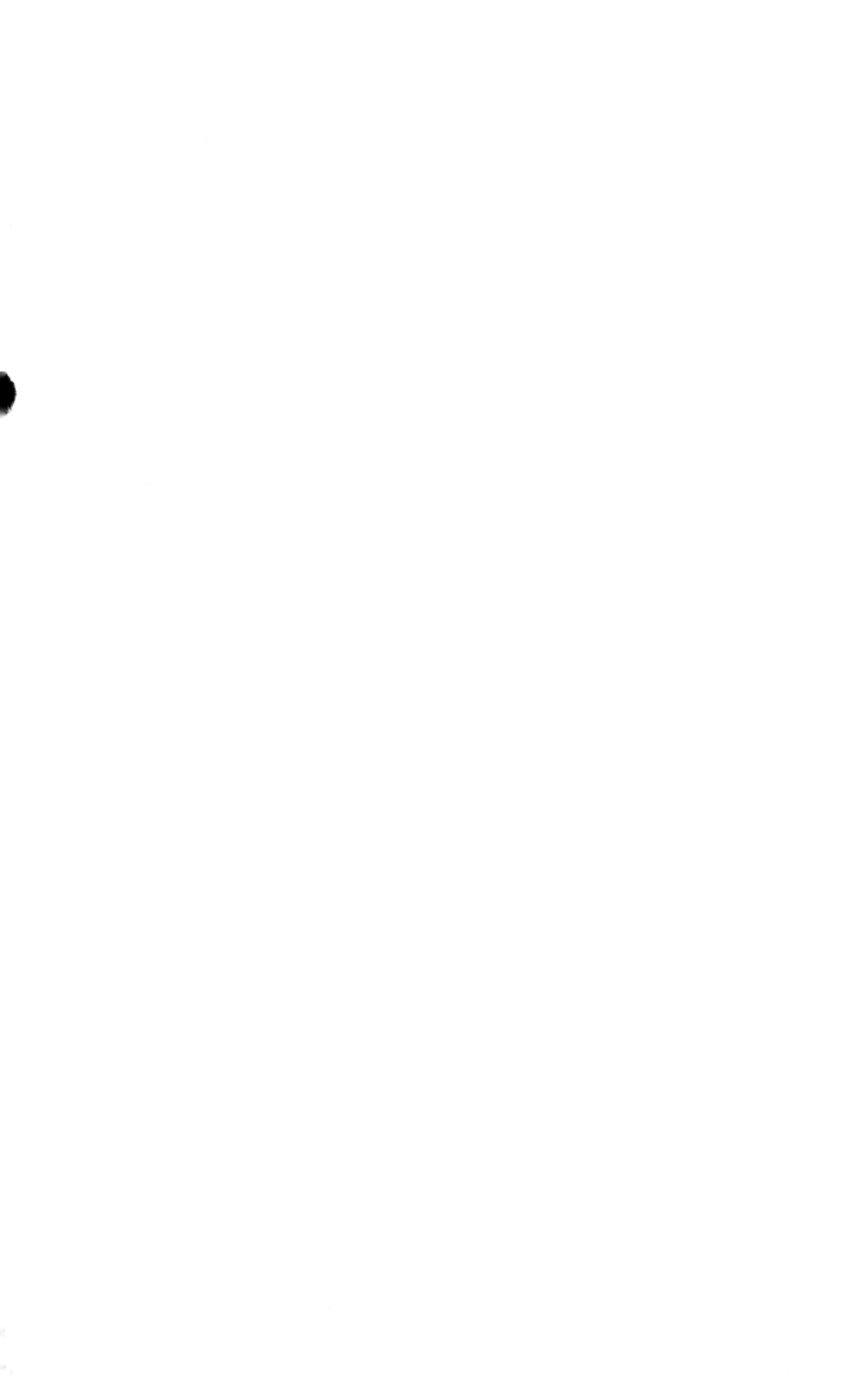

www.ingramcontent.com/pod-product-compliance
Lightning Source LLC
Chambersburg PA
CBHW050553190326

41458CB00007B/2029